Frontiers in Neuroimaging

Edited by Xianli Lv

Published in London, United Kingdom

Frontiers in Neuroimaging
http://dx.doi.org/10.5772/intechopen.105340
Edited by Xianli Lv

Contributors
Ping Xu, Zhiwei Zhou, Manikandasamy Veluchamy, Rasha Abdel-Fahim, Alwin Joseph, Chandra Jayaraman, Youtu Wu, Xianli Lv

First published in London, United Kingdom, 2024 by IntechOpen
IntechOpen is the global imprint of INTECHOPEN LIMITED, registered in England and Wales, registration number: 11086078, 5 Princes Gate Court, London, SW7 2QJ, United Kingdom

British Library Cataloguing-in-Publication Data
A catalogue record for this book is available from the British Library

Additional hard and PDF copies can be obtained from orders@intechopen.com

Frontiers in Neuroimaging
Edited by Xianli Lv
p. cm.
Print ISBN 978-1-83768-709-1
Online ISBN 978-1-83768-710-7
eBook (PDF) ISBN 978-1-83768-711-4

For EU product safety concerns:
IN TECH d.o.o., Prolaz Marije Krucifikse Kozulić 3, 51000 Rijeka, Croatia,
info@intechopen.com or visit our website at intechopen.com.

Meet the editor

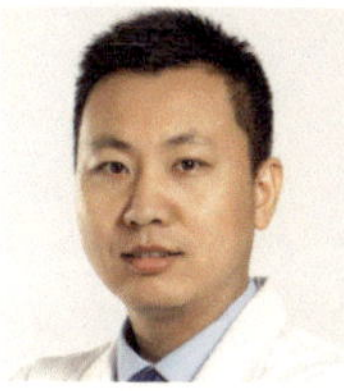

Dr. Xianli Lv, MD, is an Associate Professor of Endovascular Neurosurgery, Department of Neurosurgery, Beijing Tsinghua Changgung Hospital, School of Clinical Medicine, Tsinghua University, China. He is a deputy editor of *Neuroscience Informatics and Frontiers in Neurology*. He is also an editorial member of *Interventional Neuroradiology, Stroke and Vascular Neurology, Journal of Neuroradiology, The Neuroradiology Journal*, and *World Journal of Radiology*. Dr. Lv is a member of the World Stroke Organization (WSO) and the World Federation of Interventional Therapeutic Neuroradiology (WFITN). He was the cover person of the April 2022 issue of the *World Journal of Radiology*.

Contents

Preface

Neuroimaging has developed rapidly. Ultrasound, computed tomography (CT) scanning, magnetic resonance imaging (MRI), functional MRI, 7T MRI, and digital subtraction angiography provide high-resolution acquisitions and better contrast, making it easier to detect lesions and structural changes in brain disorders. The target disorders for neuroimaging range from tumoral diseases to vascular, neurodegenerative, and psychiatric disorders, including Alzheimer's disease, Parkinson's disease, multiple sclerosis, epilepsy, major depressive disorder, and schizophrenia. The ability of electroencephalogram and magnetoencephalogram to detect changes in brain functioning for other dementias suggests that they may also be promising biomarkers for early vascular cognitive impairment. In recent years, machine learning has had notable success in providing automated analyses of neuroimaging studies, and its role is likely to increase in the future. It is paramount for clinicians to understand these approaches, gain facility with interpreting machine learning results, and learn how to assess algorithm performance. This book presents a narrative review of these topics and an illustrative presentation of images. We expect neuroimaging to provide a new biomarker for various brain disorders.

We would like to thank all the authors for their contributions. We would also like to acknowledge the encouragement, motivation, and assistance from the Beijing Municipal Administration of Hospitals Incubating Program (PX2020039), Beijing, China and Tsinghua Precision Medicine Foundation (20219990008), Tsinghua University, Beijing, China. We are grateful to Author Service Manager Romina Rovan at IntechOpen for her dedication and hard work to ensure the smooth publication of this book. Finally, we owe a debt of gratitude to Professor Zhongcheng Wang, academician of the Chinese Academy of Engineering and the founder and pioneer of Chinese neurosurgery, for without his tireless efforts over the decades Chinese neurosurgery would not be what it is today.

Xianli Lv
Department of Neurosurgery,
Beijing Tsinghua Changgung Hospital,
School of Clinical Medicine,
Tsinghua University,
Beijing, China

Chapter 1

Introductory Chapter: Advances in Neuroimaging

Xianli Lv

1. Introduction

For over a century, scientists have been working hard to observe the living brain through the protective cover of the human skull, such as X-ray in 1918, ventriculography with contrast agent, pneumoencephalography in 1919, and cerebral angiography in 1926. The emergence of computed tomography (CT), magnetic resonance imaging (MRI), and digital subtraction angiography (DSA) has gradually replaced these examination methods [1–3]. Nowadays, a series of technologies enable researchers and clinical doctors to create stunning detailed images of our brain structure. Neuroimaging tools, including ultrasound, CT, MRI, functional MRI, DSA, positron emission tomography (PET), and single photon emission computed tomography (SPECT), play a fundamental and important role in neurosurgical and neurological treatments of brain and spine pathologies (**Figure 1**) [1–3].

2. Traumatic brain injury

Traumatic brain injury (TBI) is the main cause of morbidity and mortality worldwide [4]. Imaging plays a crucial role in the evaluation and diagnosis of TBI, particularly in its triage role in acute situations to determine which patients require emergent neurosurgical intervention [4]. The damage caused by TBI can be divided into primary and secondary mechanisms [4]. Primary injury is usually defined as direct mechanical injury caused by trauma. These injuries are usually acute and obvious, including fractures, intracranial hemorrhage, contusions, and traumatic axonal injuries [4]. This type of injury is best detected using traditional CT and MR structural imaging techniques [5].

Traumatic arterial injury can be caused by various mechanisms, including tearing caused by fracture fragments, blunt or penetrating trauma, and arterial strain [4]. The likelihood of intracranial carotid artery and vertebral artery injury is much lower than that of cervical segment injury [4]. Skull base fracture is one of the most common causes of arterial injury—the appearance of skull base fractures on CT should always prompt consideration of CT angiography (CTA) or MR angiography (MRA) for further evaluation [4]. In some cases, routine angiography may be necessary, especially when the lesion is mild or endovascular treatment is chosen (such as severe bleeding, nosebleeds, or carotid-cavernous fistula) [4]. Molecular markers have potential applications in detecting and monitoring the progression of TBI, with a particular emphasis on microRNAs as a novel molecular regulator for neural tissue damage and repair [4].

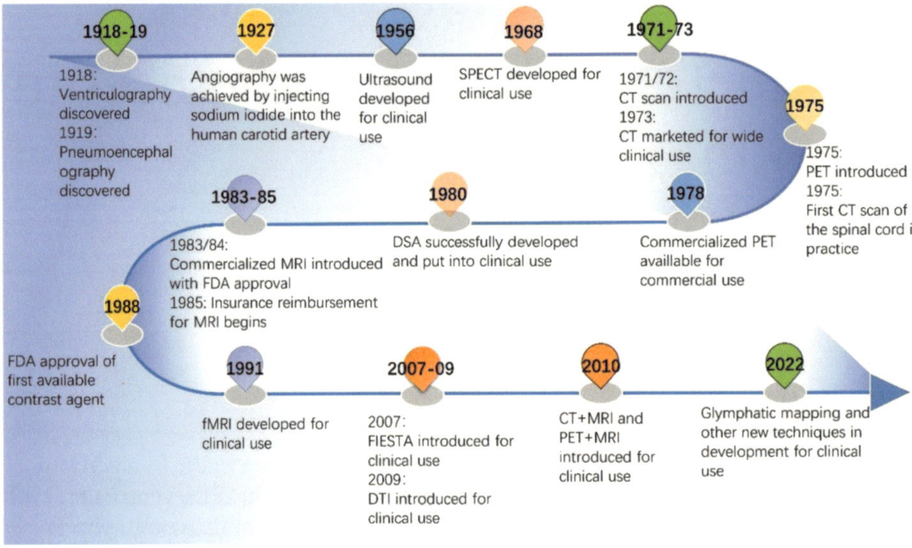

Figure 1.
The chart of the continual advancements in neuroimaging modalities.

3. Brain tumors

Neuroimaging plays a constantly evolving role in the diagnosis, treatment planning, and post-treatment evaluation of brain tumors. The MRI is commonly used in the care of brain tumor patients [5]. The use of advanced MRI sequences for structural and functional imaging (such as perfusion imaging, functional MRI (fMRI), and diffusion MRI (dMRI) sequences) provides basic information for the selection of surgical candidates, customization of personalized surgical plans based on brain structure and functional tissues, and prediction of postoperative functional outcomes [5]. Emerging radiomics techniques will be implemented to improve the diagnostic and prognostic effectiveness of neuroimaging data [5].

4. Functional neurosurgery

Accurate anatomical localization through neuroimaging techniques is crucial for achieving optimal clinical outcomes in functional neurosurgery [5]. Imaging guidance does represent the foundation of many increasingly invasive neurosurgical treatments, primarily used for the treatment of tremors and chronic pain, but has interesting prospects in the treatment of epilepsy, psychiatric disorders, and drug delivery [5]. These structural, functional, and metabolic assessments include MRI, PET, and magnetoencephalography (MEG).

The ablation of various central nervous system targets, especially deep brain stimulation (DBS), is an established tool for treating motor disorders [6]. Accurate targeting of the expected structure is crucial for optimal clinical outcomes. However, most of the targets used in functional neurosurgery are suboptimal visualized on conventional MRI. Specialized MRI sequences can usually visualize common anatomical structures in DBS surgery to a certain extent, including 1.5-T field strength [6].

The latest advances in neuroimaging, including the use of diffusion tensor imaging, diffusion tractography, fMRI, and positron emission tomography (PET), provide higher-resolution descriptions of the structural and functional connections between regions of interest [7]. In addition, new neuroimaging techniques enable DBS patients to be analyzed at the group level and delineate areas related to clinical benefits. These regions may differ from traditional target nuclei and may correspond to the center of white matter tracts or functional networks [7]. Advanced neuroimaging technology is particularly important for guiding personalized DBS-targeted treatment of refractory depression and obsessive-compulsive disorder, as the symptom characteristics and potential disorder circuits of these diseases are more heterogeneous [7].

5. Neurodegenerative disorders

Neurodegenerative diseases include Alzheimer's disease (AD), frontotemporal lobe degeneration (FTLD), Parkinson's disease (PD), and related diseases. The most commonly used neuroimaging techniques for neurodegenerative diseases are MRI and PET [8]. In neurodegenerative diseases, significant atrophy patterns on MRI are usually disease-type specific. In addition, the emergence of PET tracers targeting amyloid and tau, two major protein diseases in AD and other diseases, enables clinical trials to detect and monitor disease progression and disease-specific targeting results early on [9].

The focus of other neuroimaging studies is on psychiatric disorders, including anxiety, depression, addiction, and psychosis [9]. Recently, transcranial magnetic stimulation has been proposed as a potential pathological treatment method and biological probe for schizophrenia [9].

Non-central nervous system diseases and related treatments can have an impact on the brain and cognition. For example, non-central nervous system cancers and their chemotherapy and/or hormone therapy are associated with cognitive injury, known as cancer-related cognitive impairment (CRCI). CRCI has been proven to be associated with structural findings on MRI [10]. With the continuous development of new cancer treatment methods, the impact of cancer and CRCI treatment on brain structure, function, and cognition evaluated by neuroimaging is worth considering.

6. Cerebral and spinal vascular diseases

Intracranial aneurysms and vascular malformations are often found after intracranial hemorrhage [11]. CT scanning is the most sensitive method for detecting acute subarachnoid hemorrhage, parenchymal hemorrhage, and intraventricular hemorrhage. The display of small aneurysms on MRI is inconsistent. DSA remains the standard for fully and accurately describing patent aneurysms and arteriovenous and venous malformations (**Figure 2**).

Giant aneurysms and thrombosed aneurysms present as mass lesions, which are often detected on MRI as a screening examination [12]. MRI is usually more capable of characterizing these lesions than CT or angiography. Patients with vascular malformations with focal neurological symptoms and no bleeding are best evaluated through MRI [13]. It is easy to prove patent vascular malformations, manifested as flow void and other flow-related phenomena [14]. Hidden vascular malformations, including thrombosed arteriovenous, venous, and cavernous malformations, as well

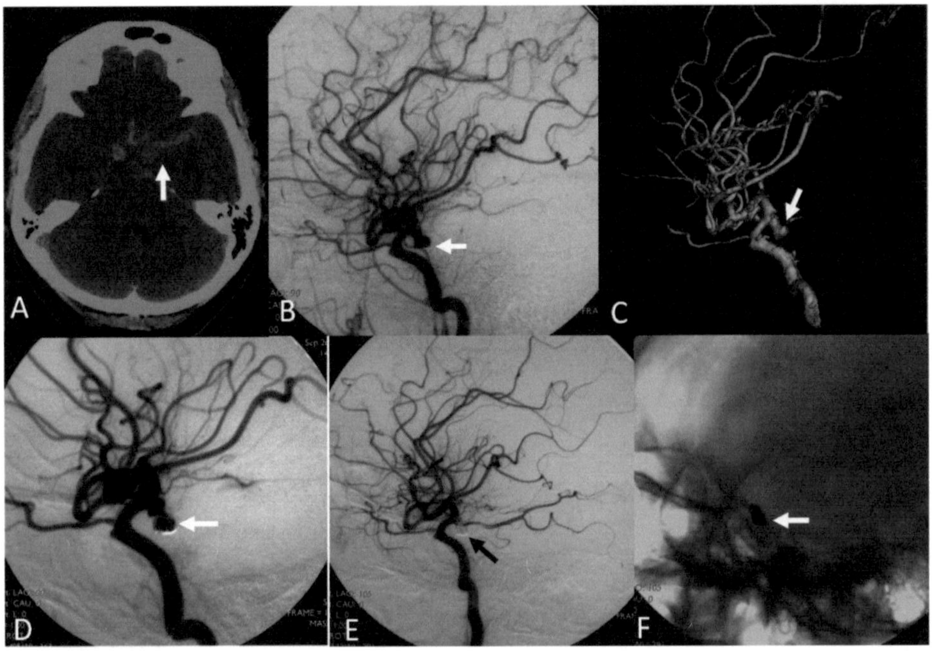

Figure 2.
A 46-year-old woman with a ruptured posterior communicating artery aneurysm was coiled. A, cranial CT scanning showing the subarachnoid hemorrhage of the left supracellar cistern (arrow). B, lateral view of the left internal carotid artery injection. C, 3-D reconstruction of the left internal carotid artery injection. Showing the aneurysm of the left posterior communicating artery (arrows). D, lateral view of the left internal carotid artery injection showing the first 3-D coil was placed into the pseudo-aneurysm (arrow). E, lateral view of the left internal carotid artery injection after aneurysm coiling showing the disappearance of the aneurysm (arrow). F, unsubtracted image showing the coil mass (arrow).

as telangiectasia, are also best detected by MRI and are not visible during angiography. The new advances in artificial intelligence and advanced imaging modes, such as PET and MRI scans, have the potential to predict early outcomes in SAH [11].

The Flow-diverter device (FDD) is a next-generation stent placed in the parent artery at the level of the aneurysm neck to disrupt flow within the aneurysm, thereby facilitating thrombus formation within the aneurysm [15]. The use of these stents is mainly suitable for unruptured aneurysms, especially aneurysms located in the internal carotid artery, vertebral artery, and basilar artery, for fusiform and dissecting aneurysms, as well as for saccular aneurysms with large neck and low dome-to-neck ratio. FDD treatment is a feasible and effective technique for unruptured aneurysms with complex anatomical structures (fusiform, dissecting, large neck, bifurcation with side branches), in which coiling and clipping are difficult or impossible [16].

Endovascular therapy has completely changed the treatment of acute ischemic stroke [17]. In the past few years, the indications for endovascular treatment have expanded to include patients receiving treatment at extended windows, such as large ischemic core infarction and basilar artery occlusion thrombectomy, as demonstrated by several randomized clinical trials [18]. Simplifying the neuroimaging protocol in the extended window to allow for non-contrast CT and CTA collaterals has also expanded the scope of mechanical thrombectomy, especially in regions around the world where advanced imaging may not be available.

7. Spinal cord tumors

FMRI of the spinal cord utilizes various methods and stimulation schemes to gain a deeper understanding of the healthy human spinal cord, laying the foundation for its clinical research and practical application [19]. New fMRI techniques and new knowledge about healthy human spinal cord have been established. Spinal cord fMRI advancement and research will further enhance our understanding of various spinal cord diseases and provide the foundation for evaluating existing and developing new treatment plans [20]. Driven by these developments, studying pathology and injury status within the spinal cord, such as fibromyalgia, multiple sclerosis, spinal cord injury, and cervical spondylotic myelopathy, have provided in-depth insights into the temporal processes of spinal cord injury and changes caused by injury, has become the next important direction in spinal fMRI.

8. Tinnitus

Although tinnitus may originate from damage to the peripheral auditory apparatus, its perceptual and painful symptoms are the result of changes in auditory, sensory, and limbic neural networks. Understanding these complex changes can promote the development of targeted therapy. When the diagnosis of Meniere's disease is unclear, a new MRI technique that can describe the maze in detail may be useful. The advancement of CT, MRI, and DSA has made diagnosis of cerebral aneurysmas, arteriovenous malformations, and dural arteriovenous fistulas possible [15, 21].

9. Conclusions

In the past few decades, neuroimaging has evolved from anatomical imaging to multimodal comprehensive anatomical and functional imaging. The minimally invasive treatment possibilities of interventional neuroradiology, image-guided laser ablation, and MRI-guided high-intensity-focused ultrasound will be used for the treatment of brain and spinal pathology.

Author details

Xianli Lv
Department of Neurosurgery, Beijing Tsinghua Changgung Hospital, School of Clinical Medicine, Tsinghua University, Beijing, China

*Address all correspondence to: lvxianli000@163.com

References

[1] Kirollos RW and Others. The history of neurosurgery. In: Kirollos R and Others, editors. Oxford Textbook of Neurological Surgery. Online ed. Oxford Academic; 1 Oct 2019. DOI: 10.1093/med/9780198746706.003.0001 [Accessed: December 27, 2023]

[2] Laing R. A history of neurosurgery. Journal of Neurology, Neurosurgery, and Psychiatry. 1998;**64**(2):284

[3] Simpson BA. A history of neurosurgery. Brain. 1999;**122**(11):2197-2199. DOI: 10.1093/brain/122.11.2197-a

[4] Smith LGF, Milliron E, Ho ML, Hu HH, Rusin J, Leonard J, et al. Advanced neuroimaging in traumatic brain injury: An overview. Neurosurgical Focus. 2019;**47**(6):E17. DOI: 10.3171/2019.9.FOCUS19652. Erratum in: Neurosurg Focus. 2021

[5] Kirkman MA. The role of imaging in the development of neurosurgery. Journal of Clinical Neuroscience. 2015;**22**(1):55-61. DOI: 10.1016/j.jocn.2014.05.024. Epub 2014 Aug 21

[6] Middlebrooks EH, Domingo RA, Vivas-Buitrago T, Okromelidze L, Tsuboi T, Wong JK, et al. Neuroimaging advances in deep brain stimulation: Review of indications, anatomy, and brain Connectomics. AJNR. American Journal of Neuroradiology. 2020;**41**(9):1558-1568. DOI: 10.3174/ajnr.A6693. Epub 2020 Aug 13

[7] Paulo DL, Bick SK. Advanced imaging in psychiatric neurosurgery: Toward personalized treatment. Neuromodulation. 2022;**25**(2):195-201. DOI: 10.1111/ner.13392

[8] Schwarz CG. Uses of human MR and PET imaging in research of neurodegenerative brain diseases. Neurotherapeutics. Apr 2021;**18**(2):661-672

[9] Buckley RF. Recent advances in imaging of preclinical, sporadic, and autosomal dominant Alzheimer's disease. Neurotherapeutics. Apr 2021;**18**(2):709-727

[10] McDonald BC. Structural neuroimaging findings related to adult non-CNS cancer and treatment: Review, integration, and implications for treatment of cognitive dysfunction. Neurotherapeutics. 2021;**18**(2):792-810. DOI: 10.1007/s13311-021-01096-5. Epub 2021 Aug 16

[11] Levinson S, Pendharkar AV, Gauden AJ, Heit JJ. Modern imaging of aneurysmal subarachnoid Hemorrhage. Radiologic Clinics of North America. 2023;**61**(3):457-465. DOI: 10.1016/j.rcl.2023.01.004. Epub 2023 Feb 19

[12] Zhang H, Liang S, Xianli LV. Intra-aneurysmal thrombosis and turbulent flow on MRI of large and giant internal carotid artery aneurysms. Neuroscience Informatics. 2021;**1**(4):100027. DOI: 10.1016/j.neuri.2021.100027

[13] Koester SW, Batista S, Bertani R, Yengo-Kahn A, Roth S, Chitale R, et al. Angiographic factors leading to hemorrhage in AVMs: A systematic review and meta-analysis. Neurosurgical Review. 2023;**46**(1):72. DOI: 10.1007/s10143-023-01971-z

[14] Sabayan B, Lineback C, Viswanathan A, Leslie-Mazwi TM, Shaibani A. Central nervous system vascular malformations: A clinical review. Annals of Clinical Translational Neurology. 2021;**8**(2):504-522.

DOI: 10.1002/acn3.51277. Epub 2021 Jan 12

[15] Lv X, Wu Z, editors. Neurointerventional Surgery: Current Status and Future Prospects. NY, USA: Nova Science Publisher; 2022. DOI: 10.52305/WOPX9620

[16] Lv X, Yang H, Liu P, Li Y. Flow-diverter devices in treatment of intracranial aneurysms: A meta-analysis and systematic review. The Neuroradiology Journal. 2016;**29**(1):66-71

[17] Samaniego EA, Boltze J, Lyden PD, Hill MD, Campbell BCV, Silva GS, et al. XIIth stroke treatment academic industry roundtable. Priorities for advancements in neuroimaging in the diagnostic workup of acute stroke. Stroke. 2023;**54**(12):3190-3201. DOI: 10.1161/STROKEAHA.123.044985. Epub 2023 Nov 9

[18] Sahoo A, Abdalkader M, Yamagami H, Huo X, Sun D, Jia B, et al. Endovascular therapy for acute stroke: New evidence and indications. JNET Journal of Neuroendovascular Therapy. 2023;**17**(11):232-242. DOI: 10.5797/jnet.ra.2023-0047. Epub 2023 Aug 29

[19] Haynes G, Muhammad F, Khan AF, Mohammadi E, Smith ZA, Ding L. The current state of spinal cord functional magnetic resonance imaging and its application in clinical research. Journal of Neuroimaging. 2023;**33**(6):877-888. DOI: 10.1111/jon.13158. Epub 2023 Sep 23

[20] Diehn FE, Krecke KN. Neuroimaging of spinal cord and cauda equina disorders. Continuum (Minneap Minn). 2021;**27**(1):225-263. DOI: 10.1212/CON.0000000000000926

[21] Raghavan P, Steven A, Rath T, Gandhi D. Advanced neuroimaging of tinnitus. Neuroimaging Clinics of North America. 2016;**26**(2):301-312. DOI: 10.1016/j.nic.2015.12.008. Epub 2016 Mar 5

Chapter 2

Preprocessing Techniques for Neuroimaging Modalities: An In-Depth Analysis

Alwin Joseph and Chandra Jayaraman

Abstract

Neuroimage analysis and data processing from various neuro-imaging modalities have been a multidisciplinary research field for a long time. Numerous types of research have been carried out in the area for multiple applications of neuroimaging and intelligent techniques to make faster and more accurate results. Different modalities gather information for detecting, treating, and identifying various neurological disorders. Each modality generates different kinds of data, including images and signals. Applying artificial intelligence-based techniques for analysing the inputs from the neuroimaging modalities requires preprocessing. Preprocessing techniques are used to fine-tune the data for better results and the application of intelligent methods. Various techniques and pipelines/workflows (steps for preprocessing the data from the imaging modalities) have been developed and followed by multiple researchers for the preprocessing of neuroimaging data. The preprocessing steps include the steps followed in removing noisy data from the inputs, converting the data to a different format, and adding additional information to improve the performance of the algorithm on the data. In this chapter, we compare the various neuroimaging techniques, the type of data they generate and the preprocessing techniques that various researchers frequently use to process data to apply them in artificial intelligence-based algorithms for the classification, prediction, and prognosis of various neurological disorders.

Keywords: neuroimaging, brain imaging, preprocessing techniques, neuroimaging modalities, neurological disorders

1. Introduction

Neuroimaging or BRAIN Imaging is a technology used to capture the brain's structure or part of the nervous system by various imaging techniques. Each neuroimaging technique has unique methods of capturing the brain's snapshot and helping doctors diagnose neurological disorders. Different techniques are used for the identification and confirmation of these neurological disorders. The doctors use multiple parameters apart from the results from the neuroimaging modalities for concluding the disease; however, the neuroimaging data plays a significant role in validating and helping the doctors to form conclusions.

Neuroimaging uses quantitative methods to concentrate on the construction and understanding of the capability of the focal sensory system, created as an objective approach to logically focus on the sound human cerebrum harmlessly. Progressively it is likewise being utilised for quantitative investigations of mind infection and mental sickness. Neuroimaging is an exceptionally multidisciplinary research field and is certainly not a clinical claim to fame.

Neuroimaging is likewise assisting us with understanding how the cerebrum creates from the outset through adulthood. Formative neuroscientists concentrate on the neurobiological underpinnings of mental turn of events. Joining utilitarian proportions of mind movement with social measures, they investigate what subtle early put-downs to the sensory system mean for mental and profound capability further down the road — for instance, the impacts of maternal ailment or youth disregard on learning, memory and consideration further down the road. Imaging devices can also take care of in the study hall: Utilising such devices, proficiency specialists have shown that an extended period of severe and deliberate perusing guidance makes the cerebrums of high-risk look capable like those of additional talented youthful people.

Making the computer learn from these imaging data and creating models that can classify and predict the symptoms of neurological disorders is challenging as imaging techniques provide data in different formats. The data passed as input for Machine Learning (ML) and Deep Learning (DL) requires significant preprocessing to understand these imaging data. Since the data generated from other imaging techniques are additional, each design has unique methods for capturing and processing data.

Current neuroimaging strategies uncover both structure and capability. They discover the cerebrum's life systems, including the honesty of mind structures and their interconnections. They clarify its science, physiology, and electrical and metabolic action. The most up-to-date devices show how various districts of the mind associate and impart. They could show with split-second timing the grouping of occasions during a particular cycle, like perusing or recalling.

For efficient data analysis, classification of the data points into categories or any such application of any data, preprocessing is an essential step in preparing data for analysis; the data from neuroimaging modalities must be equipped with the help of various preprocessing steps to make it convenient for the machines to process and analyse. Analysing and identifying the appropriate preprocessing techniques helps improve the data's applicability from the imaging techniques on ML and DL techniques. Various neuroimaging modalities and preprocessing techniques are discussed in this chapter to help understand the best practices across multiple use cases.

2. Neuroimaging modalities

Neuroimaging is the utilisation of neuroimaging innovation to gauge a part of mind capability, frequently with the end goal of figuring out the connection between movement in specific cerebrum regions and explicit mental abilities. It is an exploration device in cognitive neuroscience, mental brain science, neuropsychology, and social neuroscience [1]. Neuroimaging is a field of medication that includes utilising different strategies to envision and concentrate on the construction and capability of the cerebrum and sensory system. Several other neuroimaging modalities are used, each with novel qualities and advantages.

The neurological disorder is identified, and the doctors plan the treatment with the help of results from various neuroimaging techniques. Neuroimaging helps in gathering the structure and function of the brain. Different neuroimaging techniques used for the prognosis of neurological diseases are discussed across many research articles; [2, 3] listed various neuroimaging techniques and are mentioned in **Table 1**.

Out of the various neuroimaging techniques, the prominent neuroimaging modalities used to study the brain and its functions are the below-mentioned techniques.

1. *Magnetic resonance imaging (MRI):* MRI imaging uses a strong magnetic field and radio waves to create detailed images of the brain and other body parts. It is a non-invasive procedure commonly used to diagnose and monitor various neurological conditions.

2. *Computed tomography (CT):* CT scans use X-rays to create detailed images of the brain and other body parts. It is often used to diagnose brain injuries like concussions or haemorrhages.

3. *Positron emission tomography (PET):* PET scans use a small amount of a radioactive tracer to produce detailed images of the brain's metabolic activity. It can be used to identify brain tumours, evaluate the effectiveness of treatments for neurological disorders, and study brain function.

4. *Single-photon emission computed tomography (SPECT):* SPECT scans use a radioactive tracer to produce detailed images of brain activity. It is often used to diagnose brain likes, such as stroke and brain tumours.

Neuroimaging Techniques
Magnetic Resonance Imaging (MRI)
Functional magnetic resonance imaging [fMRI]
Positron Emission Tomography (PET)
Magnetoencephalography [MEG]
Single-photon emission computed tomography [SPECT]
Electroencephalography [EEG]
Functional neuroimaging
Transcranial magnetic stimulation
In vivo magnetic resonance spectroscopy
Near-infrared spectroscopy [NIRS]
Functional near-infrared spectroscopy
Magnetic resonance imaging of the brain
Diffusion Tensor Imaging [DTI]
Diffuse Optical Imaging
Cranial ultrasound
Computerised Tomography (CT)
Optical coherence tomography (OCT)

Table 1.
Neuroimaging techniques.

5. *Electroencephalography (EEG):* EEG measures brain activity by recording the brain's electrical activity through electrodes placed on the scalp. It is often used to diagnose epilepsy and other disorders that affect brain function.

6. *Functional magnetic resonance imaging (fMRI):* fMRI uses MRI technology to measure changes in blood flow to specific brain areas, which can indicate brain activity. It is often used to study brain function and to identify brain abnormalities.

7. *Magnetoencephalography (MEG):* MEG uses special sensors to measure the magnetic fields produced by brain activity. It is often used to study brain function and to diagnose brain disorders.

A neurological problem is a condition that influences the cerebrum, spinal rope, and nerves and can disturb the body's capabilities. Various imaging techniques mentioned above have a significant role in capturing neurological information for the prognosis of various neurological disorders. The doctors use the results from multiple imaging techniques to conclude the type of neurological disorders. Each method has a unique way of capturing imaging information from the brain; some techniques capture the magnetic activity in the brain, and electron activity, while some methods use X-rays to capture the images from the brain and to give the current overview of what is happening in the brain concerning the neurological disorder.

There are various neurological disorders; some commonly identified and researched neurological disorders [4] are listed in **Table 2**.

Out of the above-listed neurological disorders, the below-mentioned are the most commonly found and studied neurological disorders [5–11]. Various imaging techniques mentioned above are used in the diagnosis of these disorders.

- *Stroke:* Stroke occurs when blood flow to the brain is disrupted, causing brain cells to die. Strokes can cause problems with movement, speech, and other functions.

- *Epilepsy:* Epilepsy is a disorder that causes seizures and sudden bursts of electrical activity in the brain. It can cause various symptoms, including convulsions, loss of consciousness, and behavioural changes.

- *Multiple sclerosis (MS):* MS is a disease that damages the protective covering around nerve fibres in the brain and spinal cord. This damage can cause various symptoms, including muscle weakness, problems with balance and coordination, and vision changes.

- *Alzheimer's Disease:* Alzheimer's is a progressive brain disorder that causes memory loss and problems with thinking and behaviour. It is the most common cause of dementia in older adults.

- *Parkinson's Disease:* Parkinson's disease affects a person's movement. It is caused by the loss of brain cells that produce a dopamine chemical, which helps control movement.

- *Migraine:* Migraines are severe headaches often accompanied by other symptoms such as nausea, vomiting, and sensitivity to light and sound.

Neurological Disorders
Epilepsy
Parkinson's disease
Dementia
Autism
Alzheimer's disease
Brain Tumours
Cerebral palsy
Multiple Sclerosis
Stroke (Brain Attack)
Narcolepsy
Attention deficit hyperactivity disorder
Obsessive Compulsive Disorder
Migraine
Brain injury
Tourette's syndrome

Table 2.
Neurological disorders.

- *Brain injury:* A brain injury is any brain damage caused by an external force, such as a car accident or fall. Brain injuries can cause various symptoms, including problems with movement, speech, and cognition.

- *Autism:* Autism is a developmental disorder that affects communication and social interaction. It is usually diagnosed in childhood and can cause various symptoms, including difficulty with social interaction and communication, repetitive behaviours, and problems with sensory processing.

- *Tourette's syndrome:* Tourette's syndrome is a disorder that causes involuntary movements and vocalisations called tics. Tics can include eye blinks, facial grimaces, and shoulder shrugs.

Neurological disorders are not easy to be identified from other physical observations. They are closely associated with the brain, and nervous system, with a close association between nerve-related diseases and other medical conditions connected to psychiatry and mental disorders. The treatment for them can also be identified with imaging. One or more of the imaging techniques mentioned in the list of neuroimaging techniques are used to conclude the patient's neurological disorder. Disorders also share properties as they impact the patient's brain or the nervous system.

An overview of the neurological disorders, and imaging techniques used, can be deduced from **Table 3**.

Various neurological disorders and imaging techniques are discussed, and many researchers have identified and used various imaging techniques for diagnosing different neurological diseases. Different imaging techniques rule out the chances of other dementias, as many diseases share common neuro activities factors. It is evident

Neurological Disorder	Type of Imaging technique used
Alzheimer's Disease [AD]	MRI and CT are used in early-stage AD diagnosis [12]. PET and MRI are used for image analysis of AD [13]. CT and MRI have diagnostic value for AD [14].
Parkinson's Disease [PD]	MRI, PET, and fMRI are used to detect PD [15]. MRI and PET are used to identify PD early [16] MRI and its variations are widely used for PD detection [17]
Epilepsy	CT, MRI, EEG, PET, SPECT and MEG are used to detect Epilepsy [18]. MRI performs better than CT in detecting Epilepsy [19]. CT, MRI, PET, SPECT and fMRI are the modalities that can be used to detect Epilepsy [20].
Schizophrenia	DTI, fMRI, PET, SPECT, and fMRI are used to detect Schizophrenia [21].
Autism	MRI and its variations, fMRI, and DTI are the various modalities commonly used for the detection of Autism [22].
Multiple Sclerosis [MS]	MRI, PET, OCT, and other neuroimaging modalities are used for MS detection [23].
Brain Tumour	MRI and its variations, CT, SPECT, PET, and fMRI, are used to identify Brain Tumours [24].

Table 3.
Neurological disorders and neuroimaging techniques.

from **Table 3** that neurological disorders can be detected with multiple imaging techniques and the physician need to evaluate various test results to conclude the type of disorder the patient possesses.

Table 4 concludes the data type, the nature of the data and the primary technique used by the imaging technique to capture the data or the method the data is based on from the brain. The results help in planning the preprocessing strategies and processing the data for the application and study of ML and DL techniques.

The data captured from the various imaging modalities have a different structure; most have been images which doctors can quickly process. There are much preprocessing techniques and processes which are used for cleaning the data to

Neuroimaging technique	Data generated	Technique data is based on	Reference
MRI	Images	Captures pathologies, tissue properties, brain activity and blood flow velocity.	[25, 26]
fMRI	Images	Brain activity by detecting changes in blood flow.	[27]
PET	Images	The metabolic or biomedical function of tissues.	[28, 29]
EEG	Signals	Recording of the electrical activity of the brain from the scalp.	[30]
CT	Images	X-Ray images are taken from different angles and create cross-sectional images.	[31]
SPECT	Images	A nuclear imaging test using a radioactive substance and a special camera to create a 3D picture.	[32]

Table 4.
Neuroimaging techniques and the data.

remove the nose elements in them. The following section will see various preprocessing techniques specific to multiple imaging modalities.

3. Preprocessing techniques

Various preprocessing techniques are used to capture the data from the imaging technique to generate images that depict the imaging results. The imaging data is then processed to make it proper and understandable for the ML algorithms to process and extract features from these images. Mainly the preprocessing techniques help the models understand the type of neurological disorder since most diseases can be identified from the commonly used imaging techniques. Preparing the data is required to effectively process the neuroimaging data captured using various imaging techniques.

The preprocessing of neuroimaging data is an important step that is usually performed before further analysis; the preprocessing process helps the data to be effectively structured to reduce the impact of external factors and artefacts in the image. Neuroimaging data preprocessing generally involves the following steps:

- *Quality assurance:* This step involves checking the quality of the raw data to ensure that it is suitable for further analysis. This can include checking for artefacts or other issues that may affect the accuracy of the data.

- *Slice timing correction:* In functional magnetic resonance imaging (fMRI) data, the acquisition of slices may be out of synchronisation with the actual temporal sequence of the brain activity. Slice timing correction aligns the pieces to the exact time sequence of the brain activity, allowing for more accurate analysis.

- *Motion correction:* This step involves correcting for head movements or other body parts during the scanning session. This is important because activities can introduce artefacts into the data that may affect the accuracy of the analysis.

- *Spatial normalisation:* This step involves aligning the data to a common coordinate space, typically a template brain. This allows for data comparison across different subjects or sessions and can also be used to identify brain structures or regions of interest.

- *Smoothing:* This step involves applying a spatial filter to the data to smooth out noise and improve the signal-to-noise ratio. This can be useful for improving the statistical power of the analysis, but it can also introduce spatial blurring and may not be appropriate in all cases.

- *Detrending:* This step involves removing trends from the data that may be caused by low-frequency drifts or other sources of variance. Detrending can help improve the analysis's statistical power and reduce the risk of false positives.

- *Denoising/Noise Reduction:* Denoising techniques aim to remove noise and other artefacts from the data, such as motion-related artefacts or physiological noise. Denoising can be achieved through various regression-based approaches or more advanced techniques such as independent component analysis.

- *Image registration:* This technique aligns images from different acquisitions or modalities to a standard reference frame. Image registration can improve the accuracy of analysis by reducing misalignment errors.

- *Intensity normalisation:* This technique ensures that image intensity values are consistent across different acquisitions or modalities. Intensity normalisation can help correct variations in scanner performance and improve the accuracy of the analysis.

- *Skull stripping:* This technique removes non-brain tissue, such as the scalp and skull, from the images, allowing for a more accurate analysis of brain tissue.

- *Segmentation:* This technique divides the images into tissue types, such as grey matter, white matter, and cerebrospinal fluid. Segmentation can be used to create maps of brain anatomy and identify specific regions of interest.

- *Correction for head movement:* Head movement during imaging can cause misalignment of images and affect the accuracy of the analysis. Correction for head movement can be accomplished through realignment of the images or by modelling and removing the effects of head movement.

These are just a few preprocessing steps that may be performed on neuroimaging data. The measures will depend on the analysis's particular goals and the data's characteristics. Applying preprocessing techniques helps to reduce noise, enhance contrast, and correct geometric distortions. **Table 5** contains the various imaging techniques and the preprocessing techniques used concerning the imaging technique for the processing with ML and DL algorithms.

Neuroimaging technique	Preprocessing
MRI	**Noise reduction**: MRI images can be affected by various noise sources, such as electrical interference and variations in the magnetic field. Noise reduction techniques can help reduce the amount of noise in the images, resulting in more precise and accurate images. **Contrast enhancement**: MRI images often have low contrast, making it difficult to distinguish between different tissues and structures. Contrast enhancement techniques can help to increase the contrast of the images, making it easier to see the details. **Geometric correction**: MRI images can sometimes be distorted due to the complex nature of the magnetic field used to generate them. Geometric correction techniques can help correct these distortions, making images more accurately aligned with the patient's anatomy. **Registration**: MRI images of different body parts or taken at different time points can be registered or aligned, enabling comparison and analysis. **Segmentation**: MRI images often contain a large amount of data, and it can be helpful to separate different structures or tissues in the image for further analysis. Segmentation techniques can identify and extract specific structures or tissues from the images.
fMRI	**Slice timing correction:** fMRI images are often acquired in a series of slices, and the time it takes to acquire each can vary. Slice timing correction techniques can help align the slices in time, ensuring that the data accurately represents brain activity.

Neuroimaging technique	Preprocessing
	Motion correction: Movement of the head during an fMRI scan can cause artefacts in the images, making it difficult to interpret the data accurately. Motion correction techniques can help to remove these artefacts by aligning the images from different time points. **Spatial smoothing:** fMRI images often have a high noise level, making it difficult to interpret the data accurately. Spatial smoothing techniques can help reduce image noise by averaging the data over a small spatial region. **Normalisation:** fMRI data is often collected from multiple subjects, and it is essential to align the data in a shared space to be compared and analysed. Normalisation techniques can help to align the data from different subjects by transforming it into a standard coordinate system. **Detrending:** fMRI data often contains low-frequency drifts that can affect the accuracy of the results. Detrending techniques can help to remove these drifts by fitting and removing a low-order polynomial from the data.
PET	**Noise reduction:** PET images can be affected by various noise sources, such as electronic interference and variations in the radioactive tracers. Noise reduction techniques can help reduce the amount of noise in the images, resulting in more precise and accurate images. **Attenuation correction:** PET images can be distorted due to the interaction of the radioactive tracers with tissues in the body. Attenuation correction techniques can help correct these distortions, making images more accurately aligned with the patient's anatomy. **Scatter correction:** PET images can also be distorted by scattered radiation, which can cause artefacts in the images. Scatter correction techniques can help remove these artefacts by estimating and correcting for the amount of scattered radiation in the images. **Standardisation:** PET data is often collected from multiple subjects, and it is essential to align the data in a shared space to be compared and analysed. Standardisation techniques can help to align the data from different subjects by transforming it into a standard coordinate system. **Image registration:** PET images of different body parts or taken at different time points can be registered or aligned to enable comparison and analysis.
EEG	**Filtering:** EEG data often contains high-frequency noise and other unwanted signals, such as muscle activity and electrical interference. Filtering techniques can be used to remove these signals and improve the quality of the data. **Artefact correction:** EEG data can be affected by various artefacts, such as eye blinks, muscle movements, and electrical interference. Artefact correction techniques can help to remove these artefacts and improve the accuracy of the data. **Re-referencing:** EEG data is often recorded relative to a reference electrode, but the choice of reference can affect the interpretation of the data. Re-referencing techniques can change the reference of the data, making it easier to compare data from different subjects or sessions. **Epoching:** EEG data is often divided into smaller segments, or epochs, for further analysis. Epoching techniques can be used to identify and extract specific epochs of interest from the data. **Time-frequency analysis:** EEG data contains information about both the time and frequency domains. Time-frequency analysis techniques can be used to extract this information and better understand the brain's activity.
CT	**Noise reduction:** CT images can be affected by various noise sources, such as electronic interference and variations in the x-ray beam. Noise reduction techniques can help reduce the amount of noise in the images, resulting in more precise and accurate images. **Contrast enhancement:** CT images often have low contrast, making it difficult to distinguish between different tissues and structures. Contrast enhancement techniques can help to increase the contrast of the images, making it easier to see the details.

Neuroimaging technique	Preprocessing
	Geometric correction: CT images can sometimes be distorted due to the complex nature of the x-ray beam used to generate them. Geometric correction techniques can help correct these distortions, making images more accurately aligned with the patient's anatomy. **Registration:** CT images of different body parts taken at different time points can be registered or aligned to enable comparison and analysis. **Segmentation:** CT images often contain a large amount of data, and it can be helpful to separate different structures or tissues in the image for further analysis. Segmentation techniques can identify and extract specific structures or tissues from the images.
SPECT	**Noise reduction:** SPECT images can be affected by various noise sources, such as electronic interference and variations in the radioactive tracers. Noise reduction techniques can help reduce the amount of noise in the images, resulting in more precise and accurate images. **Attenuation correction:** SPECT images can be distorted due to the interaction of the radioactive tracers with tissues in the body. Attenuation correction techniques can help correct these distortions, making images more accurately aligned with the patient's anatomy. **Scatter correction:** SPECT images can also be distorted by scattered radiation, which can cause artefacts in the images. Scatter correction techniques can help remove these artefacts by estimating and correcting for the amount of scattered radiation in the images. **Standardisation:** SPECT data is often collected from multiple subjects, and it is crucial to align the data in a shared space to be compared and analysed. Standardisation techniques can help to align the data from different subjects by transforming it into a standard coordinate system. **Image registration:** SPECT images of different body parts or taken at other time points can be registered or aligned to enable comparison and analysis.

Table 5.
Neuroimaging techniques and the preprocessing.

The various preprocessing techniques used for preprocessing the different neuroimaging modalities are concluded from [33–47]. **Table 6** gives a list of various preprocessing methods used for preprocessing and organising, and enhancing data from multiple modalities for studying disorders. The preprocessing helps in better inputs for various studies by removing the noise information, improving the quality and contrast of the image and correcting the geometric and other distortions. For each imaging modality, we have to follow a different approach for the preprocessing steps; this is dependent on the process of generating the images.

Various preprocessing techniques are used to capture the data from the imaging technique to generate images that depict the imaging results. The imaging is developed with the help of various mathematical transformations and equations where the input captured by the biological process is processed. Then a final image is generated as the output, which contains the brain's current status. The preprocessing is required to make the images more efficient for analysis by removing noise, enhancing contrast, and correcting geometric distortions. The data is then processed for ML algorithms to create various models for classification and clustering. The computer learns from the images and generates an intelligent decision on the class of neurological disorder or whether the input image depicts a healthy sample or of a patient.

Neuroimage Preprocessing Techniques
Artefact Correction
Attenuation Correction
Contrast Enhancement
Contrast Enhancement
Detrending
Epoching
Filtering
Geometric Correction
Motion Correction
Noise Reduction
Noise Reduction
Normalisation
Registration
Re-Referencing
Scatter Correction
Segmentation
Slice Timing Correction
Spatial Smoothing
Standardisation
Time-Frequency Analysis

Table 6.
Neuroimage data preprocessing techniques.

4. Conclusions

Neuroimaging techniques capture brain activity for detecting and prognosis various neurological disorders. In this chapter, we have come across multiple neuroimaging techniques and neurological diseases that can be determined with the data from these neuroimaging techniques. A detailed comparison of various factors is made among the neuroimaging modalities and the diseases to identify the best practices that can be used. The various preprocessing techniques done on the data from the imaging source are also compared to determine the best preprocessing strategies that are effective for the different methods. It is essential to carefully consider which preprocessing steps are appropriate for your specific dataset and research question, as the choice of preprocessing techniques can significantly impact the analysis results.

Neuroimage preprocessing is the process of preparing neuroimaging data for further analysis or visualisation. Neuroimaging data can be collected using a variety of techniques, such as magnetic resonance imaging (MRI), positron emission tomography (PET), or functional magnetic resonance imaging (fMRI). Preprocessing of neuroimaging data typically involves steps designed to correct for various issues that can affect the accuracy of the data, such as artefacts, movements, or low-frequency drifts. The process of cleaning and preparing the data makes the data clean and adequate for analysis. Each of the neurological disorders shares various common factors. Thus, cleaning and making the process effective will help in easy and accurate results for the study.

The preprocessing techniques help in processing and transforming the data to be applied for the ML and DL algorithms to help the machines classify or cluster patient information when given to the system that can be generated. However, a detailed representation of the various techniques used will help build the preprocessing pipelines/workflows (a sequence of preprocessing techniques aligned one after the other in a sequential order for the preprocessing data from neuroimaging modalities) for the data processing [48–51]. The efficient preprocessing step needs to be identified, depending on multiple factors, including the device configuration and hardware. In future work, multiple preprocessing steps for the images can be combined, and preprocessing pipelines/workflows can be created or proposed for effective noise removal, enhancing contrast, and correcting geometric distortions.

Author details

Alwin Joseph* and Chandra Jayaraman
CHRIST (Deemed to be University), Bangalore, India

*Address all correspondence to: alwin.joseph@res.christuniversity.in

References

[1] Poldrack RA, Sandak R. Introduction to This Special Issue: The Cognitive Neuroscience of Reading. Vol. 8. Lawrence Erlbaum Associates, Inc.; 2009. pp. 199-202. DOI: 101207/s1532799xssr0803_1 [Internet] Available from: https://www.tandfonline.com/doi/abs/10.1207/s1532799xssr0803_1

[2] Wang S-H, Zhang Y-D, Dong Z, Phillips P. Neuroimaging Modalities. Singapore: Springer; 2018. pp. 13-28 Available from: https://link.springer.com/chapter/10.1007/978-981-10-4026-9_2

[3] Brain imaging techniques: Types and uses — Psych central [Internet]. Available from: https://psychcentral.com/lib/types-of-brain-imaging-techniques

[4] Neurological disorders — Johns Hopkins medicine [Internet]. Available from: https://www.hopkinsmedicine.org/health/conditions-and-diseases/neurological-disorders

[5] Cath DC, Hedderly T, Ludolph AG, Stern JS, Murphy T, Hartmann A, et al. European clinical guidelines for Tourette syndrome and other tic disorders. Part I: Assessment. European Child & Adolescent Psychiatry. 2011;**20**:155-171

[6] 9 Amazing Celebrities Diagnosed with Autism - Blogging.org Blog [Internet]. Available from: https://blogging.org/celebrities-with-autism/

[7] Headaches and Migraines - Tuggeranong Chiropractic Centre & Tuggeranong Therapeutic Massage [Internet]. Available from: https://tuggeranongchiromassage.com.au/headaches-and-migraines/

[8] Parkinsons Disease - Dr Prem Pillay [Internet]. Available from: https://www.drprempillay.org/brain/parkinsons-disease/

[9] Alzheimer's disease [Internet]. Available from: https://askjan.org/disabilities/Alzheimer-s-Disease.cfm

[10] Basics of Alzheimer's Disease and Dementia — National Institute on Aging [Internet]. Available from: https://www.nia.nih.gov/health/alzheimers/basics

[11] Questions and Answers About Stroke — National Institute of Neurological Disorders and Stroke [Internet]. Available from: https://www.ninds.nih.gov/questions-and-answers-about-stroke

[12] van Oostveen WM, de Lange ECM. Imaging techniques in Alzheimer's disease: A review of applications in early diagnosis and longitudinal monitoring. International Journal of Molecular Sciences [Internet]. 2021;**22**:1-34

[13] Reiman EM, Jagust WJ. Brain imaging in the study of Alzheimer's disease. NeuroImage. 2012;**61**:505-516

[14] Scheltens P. Imaging in Alzheimer's disease. [Internet]. 2022;**11**:191-199. DOI: 1031887/DCNS2009112/pscheltens Available from: https://www.tandfonline.com/doi/abs/10.31887/DCNS.2009.11.2/pscheltens

[15] Stoessl AJ. Neuroimaging in Parkinson's disease. Neurotherapeutics; [Internet]. 2011;**8**:72

[16] Au WL, Adams JR, Troiano A, Stoessl AJ. Neuroimaging in Parkinson disease. Journal of Neural Transmission, Supplement; [Internet]. 2019:241-248 Available from: https://www.intechopen.com/state.item.id

[17] Saeed U, Lang AE, Masellis M. Neuroimaging advances in Parkinson's disease and atypical parkinsonian syndromes. Frontiers in Neurology. 2020;**11**:1189

[18] Goodman AM, Szaflarski JP. Recent advances in neuroimaging of epilepsy. Neurotherapeutics. [Internet]. 2021;**18**: 811-826 Available from: https://link.springer.com/article/10.1007/s13311-021-01049-y

[19] Kuzniecky RI. Neuroimaging of Epilepsy: Therapeutic implications. NeuroRx [Internet]. 2005;**2**:384

[20] Brinkmann BH, So EL, Watson RE, Kotsenas AL. Neuroimaging in Epilepsy. Epilepsy [Internet]. 2021:99-116 Available from: https://onlinelibrary.wiley.com/doi/full/10.1002/9781119431893.ch7

[21] Keshavan MS, Collin G, Guimond S, Kelly S, Prasad KM, Lizano P. Neuroimaging in schizophrenia. Neuroimaging Clinics of North America [Internet]. 2020;**30**:73

[22] Wolff JJ, Jacob S, Elison JT. The journey to autism: Insights from neuroimaging studies of infants and toddlers. Development and Psychopathology [Internet]. 2018;**30**:479

[23] Cortese R, Collorone S, Ciccarelli O, Toosy AT. Advances in brain imaging in multiple sclerosis. In: Therapeutic Advances in Neurological Disorders. [Internet]. 2019. p. 12

[24] Arbizu J, Domínguez PD, Diez-Valle R, Vigil C, García-Eulate R, Zubieta JL, et al. Neuroimaging in brain tumors. Revista Española de Medicina Nuclear. [Internet]. 2011;**30**:47-65 Available from: https://pubmed.ncbi.nlm.nih.gov/21211868/

[25] Rydell J. Advanced MRI Data Processing. Linköping Studies in Science and Technology Dissertations [Internet]. 2007; Available from: http://www.imt.liu.se/Linköping

[26] MRI data analysis — Max Planck Institute for Human Cognitive and Brain Sciences [Internet]. Available from: https://www.cbs.mpg.de/former-departments/neurophysics/mri-data-analysis

[27] Logothetis NK. What we can do and what we cannot do with fMRI. Nature [Internet]. 2008;**453**:869-878 Available from: https://www.nature.com/articles/nature06976

[28] Muehllehner G, Karp JS. Positron emission tomography. Physics in Medicine & Biology [Internet]. 2006;**51**: R117 Available from: https://iopscience.iop.org/article/10.1088/0031-9155/51/13/R08

[29] Ollinger JM, Fessler JA. Positron-emission tomography. IEEE Signal Processing Magazine. 1997;**14**:43-55

[30] Al-Fahoum AS, Al-Fraihat AA. Methods of EEG signal features extraction using linear analysis in frequency and time-frequency domains. ISRN Neuroscience. 2014;**2014**:1-7

[31] Computed Tomography (CT) [Internet]. Available from: https://www.nibib.nih.gov/science-education/science-topics/computed-tomography-ct

[32] Imaging NRC (US) and I of M (US) C on the M and P of EDB. Single Photon Emission Computed Tomography. US: National Academies Press; 1996 Available from: https://www.ncbi.nlm.nih.gov/books/NBK232492/

[33] John J. Image processing techniques for identifying tumors in an MRI image. 2021; Available from: https://arxiv.org/abs/2103.15152v1

[34] Bangare SL, Patil M, Bangare PS, Patil ST. Implementing tumor detection and area calculation in MRI image of human brain using image processing techniques. Article in International Journal of Engineering Research and Applications. [Internet]. 2015;**5**:60-65 Available from: www.ijera.com

[35] LyraMaria PA. Filtering in SPECT image reconstruction. Journal of Biomedical Imaging [Internet]. 2011; Available from:. DOI: 10.5555/1992576.2043318

[36] Masutani Y, Uozumi K, Akahane M, Ohtomo K. Liver CT image processing: A short introduction of the technical elements. European Journal of Radiology. 2006;**58**:246-251

[37] Chitradevi B, Srimathi P, Professor A. An overview on image processing techniques. International Journal of Innovative Research in Computer and Communication Engineering [Internet]. An ISO 3297: 2007 Available from: www.ijircce.com

[38] Bhuvaneswari C, Aruna P, Loganathan D. Classification of lung diseases by image processing techniques using computed tomography images. International Journal of Advanced Computer Research:2277-7970

[39] Saeid Sanei, Jonathon A. Chambers. EEG Signal Processing - Google Books [Internet]. Available from: https://books.google.co.in/books?hl=en&lr=&id=f44hLefOz6UC&oi=fnd&pg=PT4&dq=EEG+image+processing+techniques&ots=FulZyriLBY&sig=9Z2CQMhswvOp7oFBZh6y3pZb3yM#v=onepage&q=EEG%20image%20processing%20techniques&f=false

[40] Xie Y, Oniga S. A review of processing methods and classification algorithm for EEG signal. Carpathian Journal of Electronic and Computer Engineering. [Internet]. 2020;**13**:23-29 Available from: https://www.degruyter.com/view/j/cjece

[41] Strecker S, Kuckertz A, Pawlowski JM. Image processing techniques for quantification and assessment of brain MRI. ICB Research Reports. Utrecht University; 2013. Available from: http://www.icb.uni-due.de/fileadmin/ICB/research/research_reports/No9.pdf

[42] Sano K. Medical image processing techniques. Keisoku To Seigyo. [Internet]. 1989;**28**:579-587 Available from: http://inis.iaea.org/Search/search.aspx?orig_q=RN:21006651

[43] Shereena VB, Raju G. Literature review of fMRI image processing techniques. In: Proceedings of the 2016 IEEE International Conference on Wireless Communications, Signal Processing and Networking, WiSPNET 2016. Presses Polytechniques Et Universitaires Romandes; 2016. pp. 1473-1476

[44] James JS, Rajesh PG, Chandran AVS, Kesavadas C. FMRI paradigm designing and post-processing tools. Indian Journal of Radiology and Imaging [Internet]. 2014;**24**:13-21 Available from: http://www.thieme-connect.de/DOI/DOI?10.4103/0971-3026.130686

[45] Madsen MT. Recent advances in SPECT Imaging. Journal of Nuclear Medicine [Internet]. 2007;**48**:661-673 Available from: https://jnm.snmjournals.org/content/48/4/661

[46] Ebrahimighahnavieh MA, Luo S, Chiong R. Deep learning to detect Alzheimer's disease from neuroimaging: A systematic literature review. Computer Methods and Programs in Biomedicine. 2020;**187**:105242

[47] Shoeibi A, Moridian P, Khodatars M, Ghassemi N, Jafari M, Alizadehsani R, et al. An overview of deep learning techniques for epileptic seizures detection and prediction based on neuroimaging modalities: Methods, challenges, and future works. Computers in Biology and Medicine [Internet]. 2021: 149 Available from: http://arxiv.org/abs/2105.14278

[48] Jaber HA, Aljobouri HK, İl Ç, Koçak OM, Algin O. Preparing fMRI data for postprocessing: Conversion modalities, preprocessing pipeline, and parametric and nonparametric approaches. IEEE Access. 2019;7: 122864-122877

[49] Preprocessing — DartBrains [Internet]. Available from: https://dartbrains.org/content/Preprocessing.html

[50] Glasser MF, Sotiropoulos SN, Wilson JA, Coalson TS, Fischl B, Andersson JL, et al. The minimal preprocessing pipelines for the human connectome project. NeuroImage [Internet]. 2013;**80**:105

[51] Park BY, Byeon K, Park H. FuNP (fusion of neuroimaging preprocessing) pipelines: A fully automated preprocessing software for functional magnetic resonance imaging. Frontiers in Neuroinformatics. 2019;**13**:5

Chapter 3

New Progress in Imaging of Pituitary Diseases

Youtu Wu

Abstract

In the last 20 years, there have been advances in imaging techniques for pituitary diseases. Magnetic resonance imaging (MRI) particularly presents high-quality structural images and the essential information needed to authorize surgery, radiation therapy, and/or drug therapy. These images can assist in monitoring long-term outcomes. Recent technological advances, such as the advent of 7-Tesla MRI, have been used for measuring tumor consistency in pituitary adenomas. Microadenomas and other pituitary incidentaloma have been more recognized in the presence of golden-angle radial sparse parallel imaging and conventional dynamic contrast-enhanced techniques. However, standard structural (anatomical) imaging, mainly in the form of MRI, acts inadequately to identify all tumors, especially microadenomas (< 1 cm diameter), recurrent adenomas, and several incidentalomas. In this respect, nuclear isotope (radionuclide) imaging promotes tumor detection beneficially. All these imaging improvements may play a central role in clinical practice, especially when considering diagnosis, differential diagnosis, or definitive intervention. They further form accurate diagnosis, advise surgery, and decrease the risk of disrupting normal pituitary function.

Keywords: pituitary, MRI, 7-tesla MRI, dynamic contrast-enhanced imaging (DCE), nuclear isotope (radionuclide) imaging

1. Introduction

The pituitary is a small endocrine gland seated in the sella turcica of the central skull base and is surrounded by the neurovascular structures of the parasellar region. The pituitary gland demonstrates many pathologies with multiple components and cell types, including neoplastic, vascular, and inflammatory processes. These conditions can affect the pituitary gland and produce endocrinologic and neurologic abnormalities. Pituitary lesions are always benign, but hypersecreted hormones or masses can seriously affect the quality of life. Therefore, early, accurate diagnosis and treatment are important. The most common lesions of the pituitary gland are adenomas. Magnetic resonance imaging (MRI) is the standard approach for evaluating the pituitary gland. Recent advances in MRI and positron emission tomography (PET) have facilitated the successful detection of tumors that may be only a few millimeters in diameter. Here, studies have indicated a prevalence rate of 3.5 to 5 times higher than previously suspected [1].

Many imaging methods focus on the diagnosis and demonstration of pituitary lesions and have already made huge progress. However, an optimal assessment has not been clarified for some occult lesions. This comprehensive review aims to discuss various updated imaging technologies regarding pituitary lesions.

2. Anatomy of the pituitary gland

Understanding the underlying anatomy depends on interpreting imaging studies of the sellar and parasellar regions. A complex neuroendocrine organ is located within the sella turcica (a cup-shaped depression in the sphenoid bone, which is also bordered anteriorly and inferiorly by the sphenoid sinus). This organ is the pituitary gland. The suprasellar cistern, which consists of the optic chiasm, is above the pituitary gland. The cavernous sinus forms the lateral walls of the pituitary fossa. It contains the sixth cranial nerve and the internal carotid arteries. It more laterally contains the third and fourth nerves. Additionally, the first and second divisions of the fifth cranial nerve sit in its walls. Anatomically, the pituitary gland is connected to the hypothalamus, which typically is via the infundibulum. Regarding embryology, the anterior and posterior pituitary lobes are distinct [2]. The adenohypophysis, the pituitary's anterior lobe, and the neurohypophysis, the pituitary's posterior lobe, emerge from embryological structures. The adenohypophysis is derived from the oral ectoderm and synthesizes multiple hormones, such as prolactin, adrenocorticotropic, thyroid-stimulating and follicle-stimulating hormones, and growth and luteinizing hormones. Arising from neural ectoderm, the neurohypophysis contains axons from the hypothalamus. It is responsible for secreting oxytocin and vasopressin. A vestigial intermediate lobe lies between the anterior and posterior lobes. The lobe is a potential site for Rathke cleft cysts [3].

Generally, the average pituitary gland is larger in women than in men. Its height is between 3 and 8 mm [4]. At birth, the size of the gland varies, when it is typically globular in shape (more so during adolescence) due to its physiological hypertrophy [5]. Yet, during pregnancy, the gland progressively develops to a large degree, where it can reach a height of up to 10 mm instantly after delivery [6]. Its size may increase in women during their 50s [6].

3. Imaging technology in pituitary and pituitary adenomas

3.1 Standard pituitary magnetic resonance imaging

Magnetic resonance imaging has brought the most advances regarding sellar and parasellar structures' radiological assessment. Magnetic resonance imaging powerfully demonstrates both normal and abnormal anatomy. It even permits detecting subtle abnormalities within an overall normally dimensioned gland. Subtle abnormalities include 1–2 mm microadenomas and infiltration/inflammation [7, 8]. The high-quality imaging of sellar and parasellar structures is critical to decision-making when radiotherapy and/or surgery are not recommended.

The pituitary gland and hypothalamus imaging have multiple potentially beneficial MRI sequences. The pituitary MRI protocol may comprise pre-contrast T1- and T2-weighted (T1W/T2W) coronal and sagittal sections with thin slices. It also should include gadolinium (Gd)-enhanced coronal and sagittal T1W images [9, 10].

Nevertheless, T1W sequences are typically used in clinical practice. They present clear contrasts between the pituitary gland and adjacent cerebrospinal fluid, blood vessel flow voids, paranasal sinus air, and bone marrow fat. T2W sequences are further utilized because their sensitivity to changes in water content can be advantageous in detecting and evaluating pituitary lesions and assessing adjacent neurological structures, such as the hypothalamus and optic chiasm. The normal anterior pituitary gland is shown to be isointense to gray matter in non-contrast T1W and T2W standard spin echo (SE) sequences. On the other hand, neurohypophysis depicts an intrinsic high T1 signal; however, it is hypointense on T2 [3, 11].

The high signal on non-contrast T1W imaging is attributed to phospholipid vesicles containing neurosecretory granules [12–14]. The absence of bright spots in the posterior pituitary may alert the clinician to the likelihood of underlying pituitary pathology; some normal subjects do not exhibit this high signal. The extent to which the posterior lobe bright spot is faint or apparent in each patient varies from scan to scan [8, 15]. Occasionally, the posterior pituitary bright spot is abnormally placed, residing in the proximal infundibulum or hypothalamus, for a commonly named ectopic posterior pituitary bright spot. This is associated with some forms of congenital hypopituitarism, specifically concerning growth hormones (GHs). There are possibly other structural abnormalities, for instance, septal hypoplasia and agenesis of the corpus callosum [16]. The position of the bright spot can also be removed with pituitary stalk interference, which is shown to follow trauma or surgical transection after damaged neurosecretory granule migration [17–19].

Intravenous injection of a paramagnetic contrast agent is a common practice and enhances the pituitary gland and stalk on T1W images. The cavernous sinuses are hypointense in relation to the pituitary gland. They are adjacent to the brain and display enhancement after contrast. The cavernous sinus's medial dural border is generally poorly visualized as a distinct structure compared with the lateral dural wall, which is more easily defined. During pituitary imaging, the naturally occurring lanthanide, Gd, is the most frequently utilized contrast agent. It changes the magnetic properties of tissues, in which it accumulates. As a result, it enhances the structure seen in MRI. Gadolinium uptake by pituitary adenomas is slower in most cases. Consequently, it triggers delayed improvement and washout characteristics. It assists in revealing a different image, especially poorly visualized microadenoma.

Gadolinium is toxic, even in its free form, and must be chelated to a carrier ligand to be permitted in clinical settings. Recently, attention has been brought to the safety of Gd-based contrast agents (GBCAs) owing to the potential for long-term central nervous system retention, typically in patients with normal renal function. As mentioned, many pituitary patients require long-term imaging surveillance with GBCAs resulting in retention of Gd in the tissues [20, 21]. Macrocyclic GBCAs show greater chemical stability compared with that of their linear counterpart. This is due to their connection with a lower risk of nephrogenic systemic fibrosis and decreased Gd tissue deposition; nevertheless, they seem to transmit a higher, albeit comparatively rare, risk of allergic reactions. Thus, while GBCAs are crucial in sellar and parasellar regions' imaging, to decrease exposure, it is essential to acknowledge when contrast agents may not be needed [22–24].

3.2 Dynamic contrast-enhanced magnetic resonance imaging

Dynamic contrast-enhanced (DCE) MRI takes a series of images over time after an intravenous contrast media. As a type of permeability imaging, it measures T1W signal-intensity changes in the process of allocating an intravenous bolus of GCBA. According to initial studies, DCE-MRI was particularly effective in detecting and precisely delineating microadenomas without contour abnormalities [25–28].

Given its intricate vascular anatomy characteristics, the pituitary gland is assured to benefit from dynamic imaging evaluation. The adenohypophysis receives most of the blood from the hypophyseal portal system supplies. The superior hypophyseal artery starts with small branches that enter the hypothalamus. It forms a primary capillary plexus. Subsequently, it transmits portal veins via the infundibulum to a secondary plexus and supplies blood to the adenohypophysis. Conversely, the neurohypophysis is supplied directly by the inferior hypophyseal artery. The inferior hypophyseal artery is an artery that branches from the internal carotid artery. Capillaries in the pituitary gland have unique fenestrations outside the blood–brain barrier, which cause the gland to strengthen with intravenous contrast administration [29].

Recent studies have proven the importance of this technique via the detection of microadenomas in patients, particularly those with Cushing's disease, with a sensitivity of 67–95% compared with that of 50–60% under conventional contrast-enhanced MRI [30–32]. Microadenomas show delayed enhancement and regression, making them more visible on DCE-MRI than conventional sequences, and a few may only appear on dynamic sequences [33]. Dynamic contrast-enhanced magnetic resonance imaging has become routine for initial imaging studies in central endocrine disorders, namely, prolactinomas, due to its negative predictive value and high sensitivity in detecting microadenomas [33]. Additionally, DCE-MRI advances surgical planning by distinguishing between normal tissue and lesions [8, 34].

Nonetheless, conventional pituitary DCE-MRI has several limitations. A trade-off happens between spatial and temporal resolutions, and the optimal parameters for collection and reconstruction are unfamiliar. Variations in slice thickness, slice interval, and imaging duration due to the absence of standardized protocols may hinder comparisons between studies and institutions. In most instances, the lack of temporal resolution hinders quantitative pharmacokinetic analysis. In the postoperative setting, conventional techniques are insufficient in fat saturation, which typically is advantageous in contrasts of hemorrhage, fat, and surgical packing material [33].

3.3 Golden-angle radial sparse parallel imaging

Golden-angle radial sparse parallel (GRASP) imaging focuses on maneuvering the restrictions posed by conventional DCE-MRI. Golden-angle radial sparse parallel imaging uses a three-dimensional gradient-echo sequence with golden-angle ordering and radial "stack-of-stars" k-space sampling [35, 36]. Conventional DCE-MRI techniques implement the acquisition of numerous images. Golden-angle radial sparse parallel imaging develops all the dynamic data by completion in a single persistent scan. First, the data is separated into sequential time frames and then recreated via an iterative method, which connects compressed sensing and parallel imaging [33, 36, 37].

This method allows the recreation of extremely under-sampled data to submillimeter isotropic resolution using a total-variation time constraint. The isotropic resolution permits multiplanar reconstruction in all time points. Golden-angle radial sparse parallel imaging may be able to distinctively permit retrospective modification of temporal resolution as high as approximately 2.5 s per frame due to the uniform distribution of the profiles in k-space. Golden-angle radial sparse parallel imaging delivers higher planar resolution, increased sensitivity to motion and flow, and improved fat suppression compared to conventional two-dimensional turbo SE examinations [33, 37]. Research on the application of GRASP imaging for pituitary imaging is in its infancy, and there are many potential avenues of research. A few published studies validate the potential of this technology to assist in managing, characterizing, and diagnosing pituitary pathology [38–41].

Golden-angle radial sparse parallel imaging has been utilized to describe the permeability features in the normal pituitary gland [40]. The posterior lobe and median eminence in normal pituitary glands show faster washin and time to the maximum enhancement than that of the anterior lobe. The median eminence and anterior lobe show faster washout than that of the posterior lobe. These results are coherent with previous DCE-MRI studies and note the gland's complex vascular anatomy [33]. Direct arterial supply to the posterior lobe allows premature improvement. The pituitary portal system, which provides the anterior lobe, is relatively slow yet proceeds in greater maximal improvement due to a stronger vascular plexus.

Golden-angle radial sparse parallel imaging illustrates in patients of subtle differences with central endocrine disturbances except morphologically normal pituitary glands. Typically, patients with GH disturbances do not have focal pituitary lesions. Golden-angle radial sparse parallel imaging has shown that in these patients, the permeability parameters of the pituitary contradict those in healthy controls [30, 40]. Particularly, the pituitary glands of hypopituitarism show fundamentally lower washin and washout in the anterior and posterior lobes. According to a prior DCE-MRI study, patients with idiopathic GH deficiency and morphologically normal pituitary glands have shown comparable permeability differences [17, 35]. For the pituitary gland, GRASP imaging permeability parameters are necessary to determine reference ranges in prospective studies with larger samples.

Golden-angle radial sparse parallel imaging aids contrasting and detecting microadenomas and cysts. Compared with the normal parenchyma of the anterior lobe, microadenomas were enhanced, albeit at a significantly lower level. Utilizing acquisitions with 20 s temporal resolution, this contrast in improvement was exposed at all time points from 60 to 140 s after contrast injection [33]. Microadenomas showed maximal enhancement at 90 ± 10 s after contrast administration, compared with that at 80 ± 10 s in the anterior lobe. In differentiating, cysts failed to enhance.

Regarding preoperative planning, GRASP imaging improves macroadenoma assessment by distinguishing normal pituitary tissue from macroadenomas [41]. Damage to the normal pituitary gland possibly impacts hypopituitarism for approximately 5% of patients during transsphenoidal resection [42]. This risk may be reduced by using preoperative imaging to localize the pituitary gland. In one study, three independent readers, a radiology resident, a medical student, and an attending neuroradiologist, localized the normal pituitary gland in patients with macroadenomas on GRASP images with an almost-perfect agreement [41]. This technique's reliability makes it an attractive option to enhance surgical planning, especially toward experience levels.

3.4 Nuclear isotope (radionuclide) imaging

3.4.1 Positron emission tomography (computed tomography/magnetic resonance imaging)

In the pituitary evaluation, the radionuclide technique has a comparatively limited role. However, some radiologists have experienced various modalities, including somatostatin receptor scintigraphy or PET, ^{18}F-fluorodeoxyglucose (^{18}F-FDG)-PET, and ^{11}C-methionine (^{11}C-Met)-PET. For instance, the ^{111}indium labeled octreotide is utilized for investigating nonfunctioning adenomas [12, 43, 44]. Yet its practicality is insufficient, as other parasellar tumors, namely, meningiomas, may express somatostatin receptors and take up octreotide [3, 45]. For assessing the biological activity of pituitary tumors, there are limited uses for PET using ^{18}F-FDG, in which most pituitary lesions are slow in growth and thus metabolically inactive. Even though the short half-life and obvious high cost of production of such pharmaceutical procedures nowadays restrict their usage for research purposes, tracers such as ^{11}C-Met have demonstrated some promise [45].

3.4.2 Somatostatin receptor scintigraphy and positron emission tomography

Within the normal human pituitary tissue, somatostatin receptors (SSTRs) are expressed in different subtypes of pituitary adenoma in varying degrees. For example, in most somatotroph adenomas, SSTR subtype 2 (SSTR2) is detectable, whereas SSTR5 expression is more changeable [46]. In managing and examining pituitary adenomas, the benefit of somatostatin receptor scintigraphy (e.g., ^{111}indiumpentetreotide) is thus complicated by certain factors: the tumor's dependence on SSTR subtype expression, the normal pituitary tissue's background uptake, and the minimal spatial resolution and sensitivity of scintigraphy when joined with single-photon emission computerized tomography [47].

3.4.3 ^{18}F-fluorodeoxyglucose positron emission tomography

There have been numerous case reports of incidental ^{18}F-FDG uptake by pituitary adenomas in the literature [48–50]. As the normal pituitary gland fails to display FDG uptake above the background activity, any significant FDG uptake generally implies pathology [51]. The usage of ^{18}F-FDG PET has been considered in various subtypes of pituitary adenoma [49, 50]. However, the findings have been greatly discouraging. For localizing corticotroph adenomas, ^{18}F-FDG PET is similar to MRI. In their retrospective study, Alzahrani et al. reported a detection rate of 58% in 12 patients who underwent conventional ^{18}F-FDG PET/computed tomography (CT) [52]. Correspondingly, ^{18}F-FDG PET still has a role in the routine management of pituitary adenomas. However, the outcome of ^{18}F-FDG PET in the identification of *de novo* and residual/recurrent pituitary adenomas is satisfactory [53, 54]. In addition, ^{18}F-FDG PET can help differentiate residual or recurrent adenoma from the remaining normal pituitary tissue because of transsphenoidal surgery once merged with ^{68}Ga-DOTATATE PET [55, 56].

3.4.4 11C-methionine PET

^{11}C-methionine PET (Met-PET) has been established to be beneficial in localizing the entire range of pituitary adenoma subtypes in terms of recurrent and newly diagnosed tumors [53, 55, 57–59], especially microadenomas [7, 55, 60]. ^{11}C-methionine PET makes the most from a substantially lower brain uptake. It not only enhances sensitivity compared with ^{18}F-FDG PE but also generates a more conductive target-to-background ratio [53, 55, 61]. Nonetheless, when Met-PET/CT is contrasted with MRI, an important limitation is the relative insufficiency of anatomical detail from CT. Thus, its capability to instruct precision surgery or radiotherapy is insufficient.

To mitigate such limitations, some groups have evaluated the importance of co-registering PET/CT and MRI images to enhance the anatomical delineation at these sites of Met-PET uptake, instruct certain treatment decisions, and assist in clinical outcomes [59, 62, 63]. Thus, the ^{11}C-Met uptake site(s) may be accurately delineated.

Gillett et al. detected that Met-PET scans ought to be normalized to the cerebellum to decrease the effects in the pituitary gland of physiological variations of the uptake of ^{11}C-Met, namely, in comparison to serial imaging. This new technique permits enhanced localization of adenomas in comparison with conventional imaging modalities, specifically because the cerebellum is utilized as the reference region. It is used between baseline Met-PET images and registered suppressed Met-PET by highlighting the regions of change. In clinical practice, implementing this technique is valuable due to definitive intervention. For example, transsphenoidal pituitary surgery or stereotactic radiosurgery is deliberated to assist targeted intervention and mitigate the liability of breaking the normal pituitary gland function. This PET/MRI generation process will eventually have minimal difficulty and be more accessible, which has been proven with various tracers [47].

3.5 7-Tesla magnetic resonance imaging in predicting the tumor consistency of pituitary adenomas

Tumor consistency is an important factor in surgical planning, as it affects resection relief and exposure to surgical operation morbidity [64–66]. Typically speaking, through the process of suction and curettage, tumors, usually with a soft consistency, are easily removed. Consistency in predicting tumors with the use of MRI is well-documented. According to T2W imaging, the hypointense tends to be associated with firmer tumors, possibly due to their increased collagen content [65, 67]. On T2W imaging, softer tumors are likely to be hyperintense, possibly in relation to much higher cystic components and/or water content [68].

Yao et al. proved that 7-Tesla (7 T) MRI could predict pituitary adenoma consistency and histopathological characteristics [66]. In the 7 T voxel-based analysis of tumor imaging, the authors demonstrated that it enabled previously inaccessible recognition of tumor heterogeneity. With permission from the ultrahigh field MRI, such techniques are facilitated by the high in-plane resolution. Moreover, the authors detected a positive correlation between tumor consistency and vascularity. With 7 T MRI, soft tumors were inclined to have a higher density of blood vessels [66].

Voxel-based particle analysis combined with 7 T MRI may be beneficial. It potentially maximizes the spatial resolution and possibly provides a more sensitive application from such use of this new imaging technique. Advanced post-processing image analysis techniques combined with 7 T ultrahigh-field MRI, for instance, the voxel-based analysis, may offer radiological tumor characterization. In such cases, they may aid in surgical decisions for the resection of pituitary adenomas.

4. Imaging technology in pituitary incidentalomas

Within the pituitary gland, pituitary incidentalomas are lesions detected incidentally in imaging for unrelated causes, such as headache, trauma, or symptoms involving the neck or central nervous system. With the wide application of imaging techniques, more and more imaging studies have found incidental pituitary tumors. The estimated prevalence of incidental pituitary adenomas is approximately 0.7/1000 (0.07%) [69].

The etiology of pituitary incidentalomas comprises many pathologies, most of which are benign adenomas. Pituitary adenomas account for approximately 90%, with most of them being Rathke's cysts, craniopharyngiomas, and meningiomas [70–72].

Magnetic resonance imaging acts as a central position in the initial evaluation. Pituitary adenomas are defined by the displacement of the pituitary stalk and perhaps deformation of the sellar diaphragm. They most commonly measure less than 1 cm and are located within the adenohypophysis. They appear to have hypointensity on the T1W series and hyperintensity on the T2W series. Nevertheless, many GH-secreting adenomas may be isointense or hypointense on T2W sequences. Many microadenomas show delayed enhancement and washout, making them more pronounced on DCE-MRI than on conventional sequences.

A few may be apparent only in dynamic sequences [9, 73]. However, compared with the normal parenchyma of the anterior lobe, microadenomas were enhanced at significantly lower levels. Golden-angle radial sparse parallel magnetic resonance imaging has excellent spatial and temporal resolutions. The potential of this technique shown in the current study was exploited in assessing the pituitary gland with an in-plane resolution of 0.7 mm, serial slice thickness of 0.8 mm, and a temporal resolution of 20 s [33]. An acquisition time of 120 s after contrast agent administration is sufficient for adequate dynamic assessment of the pituitary gland, optimizing scan time using the magnet.

In contrast to conventional dynamic MRI techniques that accomplish multiple separate exams, GRASP technology acquires all dynamic information in a single sequential scan where contrast agent injection occurs. Image reconstruction is later achieved by merging the data into consecutive time frames and reconstructing the frames using an iterative method combining parallel imaging and compressed sensing [36, 40]. Therefore, GRASP provides higher planar resolution, increased sensitivity to motion and flow, and improved fat suppression compared to conventional two-dimensional turbo-SE examinations [74]. Rathke's cysts are the most generally known cystic pituitary incidentalomas, and MRI findings depend on the cyst's contents. Rathke's cysts are commonly hyperintense on T1W imaging with characteristic T2 hypointense intra-cystic nodules. In most cases, the cyst wall fails to enhance following contrast administration [75, 76]. The appearance of craniopharyngiomas on MRI also depends on the content of the cyst, the proportion of solid components, and the probable presence of calcifications. Their solid portion is commonly iso- or hypointense on T1 and hyperintense on T2, whereas the cystic portion is hyperintense on T1W sequences. Calcified tumors are characteristic. Rim and nodular calcifications are greatly identified on CT [77].

5. Imaging technology in primary hypophysitis and immunotherapy-related hypophysitis

The classification of primary hypophysitis includes plasmacytic, granulomatous, lymphocytic, xanthomatous, or mixed [78]. Generally, they are nearly identical to immunotherapy-associated hypophysitis (IH) and share the same radiographic features. Immunotherapy-associated hypophysitis is a generally known immune-related adverse event that happens most frequently with regimens comprising cytotoxic T-lymphocyte antigen 4 suppression, especially ipilimumab. The MRI plays a crucial role in diagnosing hypophysitis. And 2-[^{18}F]-fluoro-2-deoxy-D-glucose PET/CT gives complementary diagnostic information.

For primary hypophysitis and IH, the key feature of MRI is the diffuse and transient enlargement of the pituitary gland, which is always modest [79, 80]. The absolute peak size shown in the study of the pituitary gland was 2 cm in 59 patients with IH. In primary hypophysitis and IH, the posterior pituitary bright spot with connected infundibular/suprasellar abnormality appears absent in the MRI. Lesions are, for the most part, T1 isointense. Usually, they improve markedly on contrast T1W imaging [81]. Homogeneous pituitary enhancement is often accompanied by hypophysitis, and other pituitary lesions often accompany heterogeneous enhancement. Pituitary stalk thickening is seen in IH in 59% of the cases [80]. Immunotherapy-associated hypophysitis causes a transient increase in pituitary size, which generally resolves within several months. In terms of monitoring IH, FDG-PET/CT holds value [79]. The normal pituitary gland fails to exhibit FDG uptake above background activity, so any significant FDG uptake usually demonstrates pathology. However, the pituitary should be monitored exclusively during the FDG-PET/CT studies routinely performed after initiating an immune checkpoint inhibitor (ICI) to determine the pathological uptake. In the case of longitudinal imaging, PET can individualize hypophysitis from neoplastic lesions, such as metastases or macroadenomas [82]. After ICI initiation, transient pituitary FDG hypermetabolism is a common sign of IH [79]. The insufficiency of FDG uptake in sellar lesions also aids in characterization, advising non-neoplastic pathology, such as Rathke's cleft cyst or a microadenoma (approximately half do not demonstrate FDG uptake) [83].

6. Conclusion

Imaging examination is indispensable in diagnosing and managing pituitary lesions, especially MRI. With the understanding of such lesions, there is a higher demand for the development of imaging technology. New evaluation methods have been adopted for diagnosing pituitary microadenoma, pituitary incidentaloma, hypophysitis, and recurrent pituitary tumors, such as 7 T MRI, DCE imaging, and nuclear isotope imaging. With the progress of technology, more new technologies will be available to assess diagnosis and treatment options.

Conflict of interest

The author declares no conflict of interest.

Author details

Youtu Wu
Neurosurgical Department, Beijing Tsinghua Changgung Hospital, Beijing, People's Republic of China

*Address all correspondence to: wuyoutu@sina.com

References

[1] Vandeva S, Jaffrain-Rea ML, Daly AF, Tichomirowa M, Zacharieva S, Beckers A. The genetics of pituitary adenomas. Best Practice & Research. Clinical Endocrinology & Metabolism. 2010;**24**(3):461-476. DOI: 10.1016/j.beem.2010.03.001

[2] Elster AD. Modern imaging of the pituitary. Radiology. 1993;**187**(1):1-14. DOI: 10.1148/radiology.187.1.8451394

[3] Shah S, Waldman AD, Mehta A. Advances in pituitary imaging technology and future prospects. Best Practice & Research. Clinical Endocrinology & Metabolism. 2012;**26**(1):35-46. DOI: 10.1016/j.beem.2011.08.003

[4] Denk CC, Onderoglu S, Ilgi S, Gurcan F. Height of normal pituitary gland on MRI: Differences between age groups and sexes. Okajimas Folia Anatomica Japonica. 1999;**76**(2-3):81-87. DOI: 10.2535/ofaj1936.76.2-3_81

[5] Saba M, Ebrahimi HA, Ahmadi-Pour H, Khodadoust M. Height, shape and anterior-posterior diameter of pituitary gland on magnetic resonance imaging among patients with multiple sclerosis compared to normal individuals. Iran Journal of Neurology. 2017;**16**(4):218-220

[6] Dinc H, Esen F, Demirci A, Sari A, Resit GH. Pituitary dimensions and volume measurements in pregnancy and post partum. MR assessment. Acta Radiology. 1998;**39**(1):64-69. DOI: 10.1080/02841859809172152

[7] MacFarlane J, Bashari WA, Senanayake R, Gillett D, van der Meulen M, Powlson AS, et al. Advances in the imaging of pituitary Tumors. Endocrinology and Metabolism Clinics of North America. 2020;**49**(3):357-373. DOI: 10.1016/j.ecl.2020.06.002

[8] Bashari WA, Senanayake R, Fernandez-Pombo A, Gillett D, Koulouri O, Powlson AS, et al. Modern imaging of pituitary adenomas. Best Practice & Research. Clinical Endocrinology & Metabolism. 2019;**33**(2):101278. DOI: 10.1016/j.beem.2019.05.002

[9] Paschou SA, Vryonidou A, Goulis DG. Pituitary incidentalomas: A guide to assessment, treatment and follow-up. Maturitas. 2016;**92**:143-149. DOI: 10.1016/j.maturitas.2016.08.006

[10] Vasilev V, Rostomyan L, Daly AF, Potorac I, Zacharieva S, Bonneville JF, et al. MANAGEMENT OF ENDOCRINE DISEASE: Pituitary 'incidentaloma': neuroradiological assessment and differential diagnosis. European Journal of Endocrinology. 2016;**175**(4):R171-R184. DOI: 10.1530/EJE-15-1272

[11] Klyn V, Dekeyzer S, Van Eetvelde R, Roels P, Vergauwen O, Devolder P, et al. Presence of the posterior pituitary bright spot sign on MRI in the general population: A comparison between 1.5 and 3T MRI and between 2D-T1 spin-echo- and 3D-T1 gradient-echo sequences. Pituitary. 2018;**21**(4):379-383. DOI: 10.1007/s11102-018-0885-3

[12] Bashari WA, Senanayake R, MacFarlane J, Gillett D, Powlson AS, Kolias A, et al. Using molecular imaging to enhance decision making in the management of pituitary adenomas. Journal of Nuclear Medicine. 2021;**62**(Suppl. 2):57S-62S. DOI: 10.2967/jnumed.120.251546

[13] Kucharczyk W, Lenkinski RE, Kucharczyk J, Henkelman RM. The effect of phospholipid vesicles on the NMR relaxation of water: An explanation for the MR appearance of the neurohypophysis? AJNR. American Journal of Neuroradiology. 1990;**11**(4):693-700

[14] Kucharczyk W, Crawley AP, Kelly WM, Henkelman RM. Effect of multislice interference on image contrast in T2- and T1-weighted MR images. AJNR. American Journal of Neuroradiology. 1988;**9**(3):443-451

[15] Brooks BS, el Gammal T, Allison JD, Hoffman WH. Frequency and variation of the posterior pituitary bright signal on MR images. AJNR. American Journal of Neuroradiology. 1989;**10**(5):943-948

[16] Argyropoulou MI, Kiortsis DN. MRI of the hypothalamic-pituitary axis in children. Pediatric Radiology. 2005;**35**(11):1045-1055. DOI: 10.1007/s00247-005-1512-9

[17] Wang S, Xiao D, Lin K, Zhao L, Wei L. Magnetic resonance imaging characteristics of residual pituitary tissues following transsphenoidal resection of pituitary macroadenomas. Neurology India. 2021;**69**(4):867-873. DOI: 10.4103/0028-3886.325377

[18] Meyrignac O, Idir IS, Cognard C, Bonneville JF, Bonneville F. 3D TOF MR angiography to depict pituitary bright spot and to detect posterior pituitary lobe cyst: Original description at 3T MR imaging. Journal of Neuroradiology. 2015;**42**(6):321-325. DOI: 10.1016/j.neurad.2015.04.009

[19] Saeki N, Tokunaga H, Wagai N, Sunami K, Murai H, Kubota M, et al. MRI of ectopic posterior pituitary bright spot with large adenomas: Appearances and relationship to transient postoperative diabetes insipidus. Neuroradiology. 2003;**45**(10):713-716. DOI: 10.1007/s00234-003-1018-9

[20] Nachtigall LB, Karavitaki N, Kiseljak-Vassiliades K, Ghalib L, Fukuoka H, Syro LV, et al. Physicians' awareness of gadolinium retention and MRI timing practices in the longitudinal management of pituitary tumors: A "Pituitary Society" survey. Pituitary. 2019;**22**(1):37-45. DOI: 10.1007/s11102-018-0924-0

[21] Lersy F, Boulouis G, Clement O, Desal H, Anxionnat R, Berge J, et al. Consensus Guidelines of the French Society of Neuroradiology (SFNR) on the use of Gadolinium-Based Contrast agents (GBCAs) and related MRI protocols in neuroradiology. Journal of Neuroradiology. 2020;**47**(6):441-449. DOI: 10.1016/j.neurad.2020.05.008

[22] Rudnick MR, Wahba IM, Leonberg-Yoo AK, Miskulin D, Litt HI. Risks and options with gadolinium-based contrast agents in patients with CKD: A review. American Journal of Kidney Diseases. 2021;**77**(4):517-528. DOI: 10.1053/j.ajkd.2020.07.012

[23] Bonneville JF. A plea for the T2W MR sequence for pituitary imaging. Pituitary. 2019;**22**(2):195-197. DOI: 10.1007/s11102-018-0928-9

[24] Costelloe CM, Amini B, Madewell JE. Risks and benefits of gadolinium-based contrast-enhanced MRI. Seminars in Ultrasound, CT, and MR. 2020;**41**(2):170-182. DOI: 10.1053/j.sult.2019.12.005

[25] Maier C, Riedl M, Clodi M, Bieglmayer C, Mlynarik V, Trattnig S, et al. Dynamic contrast-enhanced MR imaging of the stimulated pituitary gland. NeuroImage. 2004;**22**(1):347-352. DOI: 10.1016/j.neuroimage.2004.01.006

[26] Gao R, Isoda H, Tanaka T, Inagawa S, Takeda H, Takehara Y, et al. Dynamic gadolinium-enhanced MR imaging of pituitary adenomas: Usefulness of sequential sagittal and coronal plane images. European Journal of Radiology. 2001;**39**(3):139-146. DOI: 10.1016/s0720-048x(01)00354-0

[27] Kamimura K, Nakajo M, Yoneyama T, Bohara M, Nakanosono R, Fujio S, et al. Quantitative pharmacokinetic analysis of high-temporal-resolution dynamic contrast-enhanced MRI to differentiate the normal-appearing pituitary gland from pituitary macroadenoma. Japanese Journal of Radiology. 2020;**38**(7):649-657. DOI: 10.1007/s11604-020-00942-4

[28] Elster AD. High-resolution, dynamic pituitary MR imaging: Standard of care or academic pastime? AJR. American Journal of Roentgenology. 1994;**163**(3):680-682. DOI: 10.2214/ajr.163.3.8079867

[29] Chapman PR, Singhal A, Gaddamanugu S, Prattipati V. Neuroimaging of the pituitary gland: Practical anatomy and pathology. Radiologic Clinics of North America. 2020;**58**(6):1115-1133. DOI: 10.1016/j.rcl.2020.07.009

[30] Vitale G, Tortora F, Baldelli R, Cocchiara F, Paragliola RM, Sbardella E, et al. Pituitary magnetic resonance imaging in Cushing's disease. Endocrine. 2017;**55**(3):691-696. DOI: 10.1007/s12020-016-1038-y

[31] Liu Z, Zhang X, Wang Z, You H, Li M, Feng F, et al. High positive predictive value of the combined pituitary dynamic enhanced MRI and high-dose dexamethasone suppression tests in the diagnosis of Cushing's disease bypassing bilateral inferior petrosal sinus sampling. Scientific Reports. 2020;**10**(1):14694. DOI: 10.1038/s41598-020-71628-0

[32] Tabarin A, Laurent F, Catargi B, Olivier-Puel F, Lescene R, Berge J, et al. Comparative evaluation of conventional and dynamic magnetic resonance imaging of the pituitary gland for the diagnosis of Cushing's disease. Clinical Endocrinology. 1998;**49**(3):293-300. DOI: 10.1046/j.1365-2265.1998.00541.x

[33] Lee MD, Young MG, Fatterpekar GM. "The Pituitary within GRASP"—Golden-angle radial sparse parallel dynamic MRI technique and applications to the pituitary gland. Seminars in Ultrasound, CT, and MR. 2021;**42**(3):307-315. DOI: 10.1053/j.sult.2021.04.007

[34] Taheri MS, Ghomi Z, Mirshahi R, Moradpour M, Niroomand M, Yarmohamadi P, et al. Usefulness of subtraction images for accurate diagnosis of pituitary microadenomas in dynamic contrast-enhanced magnetic resonance imaging. Acta Radiologica. 2022;**2022**:284. DOI: 10.1177/02841851221107344

[35] Winkelmann S, Schaeffter T, Koehler T, Eggers H, Doessel O. An optimal radial profile order based on the Golden Ratio for time-resolved MRI. IEEE Transactions on Medical Imaging. 2007;**26**(1):68-76. DOI: 10.1109/TMI.2006.885337

[36] Chandarana H, Feng L, Block TK, Rosenkrantz AB, Lim RP, Babb JS, et al. Free-breathing contrast-enhanced multiphase MRI of the liver using a combination of compressed sensing, parallel imaging, and golden-angle radial sampling. Investigative Radiology. 2013;**48**(1):10-16. DOI: 10.1097/RLI.0b013e318271869c

[37] Otazo R, Kim D, Axel L, Sodickson DK. Combination of compressed sensing and parallel imaging for highly accelerated first-pass cardiac perfusion MRI. Magnetic Resonance in

Medicine. 2010;**64**(3):767-776. DOI: 10.1002/mrm.22463

[38] Hainc N, Stippich C, Reinhardt J, Stieltjes B, Blatow M, Mariani L, et al. Golden-angle radial sparse parallel (GRASP) MRI in clinical routine detection of pituitary microadenomas: First experience and feasibility. Magnetic Resonance Imaging. 2019;**60**:38-43. DOI: 10.1016/j.mri.2019.03.015

[39] Huang L, Fatterpekar G, Charles S, Golub D, Zagzag D, Agrawal N. Clinical course and unique features of silent corticotroph adenomas. World Neurosurgery. 2022;**161**:e274-ee81. DOI: 10.1016/j.wneu.2022.01.119

[40] Rossi Espagnet MC, Bangiyev L, Haber M, Block KT, Babb J, Ruggiero V, et al. High-resolution DCE-MRI of the pituitary gland using radial k-space acquisition with compressed sensing reconstruction. AJNR. American Journal of Neuroradiology. 2015;**36**(8):1444-1449. DOI: 10.3174/ajnr.A4324

[41] Sen R, Sen C, Pack J, Block KT, Golfinos JG, Prabhu V, et al. Role of high-resolution dynamic contrast-enhanced MRI with Golden-angle radial sparse parallel reconstruction to identify the Normal pituitary gland in patients with macroadenomas. AJNR. American Journal of Neuroradiology. 2017;**38**(6):1117-1121. DOI: 10.3174/ajnr.A5244

[42] Fatemi N, Dusick JR, Mattozo C, McArthur DL, Cohan P, Boscardin J, et al. Pituitary hormonal loss and recovery after transsphenoidal adenoma removal. Neurosurgery. 2008;**63**(4):709-718. DOI: 10.1227/01.NEU.0000325725.77132.90

[43] Challis BG, Powlson AS, Casey RT, Pearson C, Lam BY, Ma M, et al. Adult-onset hyperinsulinaemic hypoglycaemia in clinical practice: Diagnosis, aetiology and management. Endocrine Connections. 2017;**6**(7):540-548. DOI: 10.1530/EC-17-0076

[44] Tjornstrand A, Casar-Borota O, Heurling K, Scholl M, Gjertsson P, Himmelman J, et al. Lower (68) Ga-DOTATOC uptake in nonfunctioning pituitary neuroendocrine tumours compared to normal pituitary gland-A proof-of-concept study. Clinical Endocrinology. 2020;**92**(3):222-231. DOI: 10.1111/cen.14144

[45] Khan S, Lloyd C, Szyszko T, Win Z, Rubello D, Al-Nahhas A. PET imaging in endocrine tumours. Minerva Endocrinologica. 2008;**33**(2):41-52

[46] Nielsen S, Mellemkjaer S, Rasmussen LM, Ledet T, Olsen N, Bojsen-Moller M, et al. Expression of somatostatin receptors on human pituitary adenomas in vivo and ex vivo. Journal of Endocrinological Investigation. 2001;**24**(6):430-437. DOI: 10.1007/BF03351043

[47] Wang H, Hou B, Lu L, Feng M, Zang J, Yao S, et al. PET/MRI in the diagnosis of hormone-producing pituitary microadenoma: A prospective pilot study. Journal of Nuclear Medicine. 2018;**59**(3):523-528. DOI: 10.2967/jnumed.117.191916

[48] Joshi P, Lele V, Gandhi R. Incidental detection of clinically occult follicle stimulating hormone secreting pituitary adenoma on whole body 18-Fluorodeoxyglucose positron emission tomography-computed tomography. Indian Journal of Nuclear Medicine. 2011;**26**(1):34-35. DOI: 10.4103/0972-3919.84611

[49] Ding Y, Wu S, Xu J, Wang H, Ma C. Pituitary 18F-FDG uptake correlates with serum TSH levels in thyroid cancer patients on 18F-FDG PET/CT.

Nuclear Medicine Communications. 2019;**40**(1):57-62. DOI: 10.1097/MNM.0000000000000940

[50] Zhou J, Ju H, Zhu L, Pan Y, Lv J, Zhang Y. Value of fluorine-18-fluorodeoxyglucose PET/CT in localizing the primary lesion in adrenocorticotropic hormone-dependent Cushing syndrome. Nuclear Medicine Communications. 2019;**40**(5):539-544. DOI: 10.1097/MNM.0000000000000989

[51] Jeong SY, Lee SW, Lee HJ, Kang S, Seo JH, Chun KA, et al. Incidental pituitary uptake on whole-body 18F-FDG PET/CT: A multicentre study. European Journal of Nuclear Medicine and Molecular Imaging. 2010;**37**(12):2334-2343. DOI: 10.1007/s00259-010-1571-5

[52] Alzahrani AS, Farhat R, Al-Arifi A, Al-Kahtani N, Kanaan I, Abouzied M. The diagnostic value of fused positron emission tomography/computed tomography in the localization of adrenocorticotropin-secreting pituitary adenoma in Cushing's disease. Pituitary. 2009;**12**(4):309-314. DOI: 10.1007/s11102-009-0180-4

[53] Iglesias P, Cardona J, Diez JJ. The pituitary in nuclear medicine imaging. European Journal of Internal Medicine. 2019;**68**:6-12. DOI: 10.1016/j.ejim.2019.08.008

[54] Seok H, Lee EY, Choe EY, Yang WI, Kim JY, Shin DY, et al. Analysis of 18F-fluorodeoxyglucose positron emission tomography findings in patients with pituitary lesions. The Korean Journal of Internal Medicine. 2013;**28**(1):81-88. DOI: 10.3904/kjim.2013.28.1.81

[55] Feng Z, He D, Mao Z, Wang Z, Zhu Y, Zhang X, et al. Utility of 11C-methionine and 18F-FDG PET/CT in patients with functioning pituitary adenomas. Clinical Nuclear Medicine. 2016;**41**(3):e130-e134. DOI: 10.1097/RLU.0000000000001085

[56] Zhao X, Xiao J, Xing B, Wang R, Zhu Z, Li F. Comparison of (68)Ga DOTATATE to 18F-FDG uptake is useful in the differentiation of residual or recurrent pituitary adenoma from the remaining pituitary tissue after transsphenoidal adenomectomy. Clinical Nuclear Medicine. 2014;**39**(7):605-608. DOI: 10.1097/RLU.0000000000000457

[57] Zhang F, He Q, Luo G, Long Y, Li R, Ding L, et al. The combination of (13)N-ammonia and (11)C-methionine in differentiation of residual/recurrent pituitary adenoma from the pituitary gland remnant after trans-sphenoidal Adenomectomy. BMC Cancer. 2021;**21**(1):837. DOI: 10.1186/s12885-021-08574-1

[58] Bashari WA, van der Meulen M, MacFarlane J, Gillett D, Senanayake R, Serban L, et al. (11)C-methionine PET aids localization of microprolactinomas in patients with intolerance or resistance to dopamine agonist therapy. Pituitary. 2022;**25**(4):573-586. DOI: 10.1007/s11102-022-01229-9

[59] Koulouri O, Steuwe A, Gillett D, Hoole AC, Powlson AS, Donnelly NA, et al. A role for 11C-methionine PET imaging in ACTH-dependent Cushing's syndrome. European Journal of Endocrinology. 2015;**173**(4):M107-M120. DOI: 10.1530/EJE-15-0616

[60] Berkmann S, Roethlisberger M, Mueller B, Christ-Crain M, Mariani L, Nitzsche E, et al. Selective resection of cushing microadenoma guided by preoperative hybrid 18-fluoroethyl-L-tyrosine and 11-C-methionine PET/MRI. Pituitary. 2021;**24**(6):878-886. DOI: 10.1007/s11102-021-01160-5

[61] Tomura N, Saginoya T, Mizuno Y, Goto H. Accumulation of (11) C-methionine in the normal pituitary gland on (11)C-methionine PET. Acta Radiologica. 2017;**58**(3):362-366. DOI: 10.1177/0284185116651005

[62] Koulouri O, Kandasamy N, Hoole AC, Gillett D, Heard S, Powlson AS, et al. Successful treatment of residual pituitary adenoma in persistent acromegaly following localisation by 11C-methionine PET co-registered with MRI. European Journal of Endocrinology. 2016;**175**(5):485-498. DOI: 10.1530/EJE-16-0639

[63] Rodriguez-Barcelo S, Gutierrez-Cardo A, Dominguez-Paez M, Medina-Imbroda J, Romero-Moreno L, Arraez-Sanchez M. Clinical usefulness of coregistered 11C-methionine positron emission tomography/3-T magnetic resonance imaging at the follow-up of acromegaly. World Neurosurgery. 2014;**82**(3-4):468-473. DOI: 10.1016/j.wneu.2013.11.011

[64] Ding W, Huang Z, Zhou G, Li L, Zhang M, Li Z. Diffusion-weighted imaging for predicting tumor consistency and extent of resection in patients with pituitary adenoma. Neurosurgical Review. 2021;**44**(5):2933-2941. DOI: 10.1007/s10143-020-01469-y

[65] Sitthinamsuwan B, Khampalikit I, Nunta-aree S, Srirabheebhat P, Witthiwej T, Nitising A. Predictors of meningioma consistency: A study in 243 consecutive cases. Acta Neurochirurgica. 2012;**154**(8):1383-1389. DOI: 10.1007/s00701-012-1427-9

[66] Yao A, Rutland JW, Verma G, Banihashemi A, Padormo F, Tsankova NM, et al. Pituitary adenoma consistency: Direct correlation of ultrahigh field 7T MRI with histopathological analysis. European Journal of Radiology. 2020;**126**:108931. DOI: 10.1016/j.ejrad.2020.108931

[67] Smith KA, Leever JD, Chamoun RB. Predicting consistency of meningioma by magnetic resonance imaging. Journal of Neurological Surgery B Skull Base. 2015;**76**(3):225-229. DOI: 10.1055/s-0034-1543965

[68] Winter F, Furtner J, Pleyel A, Woehrer A, Callegari K, Hosmann A, et al. How to predict the consistency and vascularity of meningiomas by MRI: An institutional experience. Neurological Research. 2021;**43**(8):693-699. DOI: 10.1080/01616412.2021.1922171

[69] Fernandez A, Karavitaki N, Wass JA. Prevalence of pituitary adenomas: A community-based, cross-sectional study in Banbury (Oxfordshire, UK). Clinical Endocrinology. 2010;**72**(3):377-382. DOI: 10.1111/j.1365-2265.2009.03667.x

[70] Tresoldi AS, Carosi G, Betella N, Del Sindaco G, Indirli R, Ferrante E, et al. Clinically nonfunctioning pituitary incidentalomas: Characteristics and natural history. Neuroendocrinology. 2020;**110**(7-8):595-603. DOI: 10.1159/000503256

[71] Lania A, Beck-Peccoz P. Pituitary incidentalomas. Best Practice & Research. Clinical Endocrinology & Metabolism. 2012;**26**(4):395-403. DOI: 10.1016/j.beem.2011.10.009

[72] Giraldi E, Allen JW, Ioachimescu AG. Pituitary incidentalomas: Best practices and looking ahead. Endocrine Practice. 2023;**29**(1):60-68. DOI: 10.1016/j.eprac.2022.10.004

[73] Karimian-Jazi K. Pituitary gland tumors. Der Radiologe. 2019;**59**(11):982-991. DOI: 10.1007/s00117-019-0570-1

[74] Feng L, Grimm R, Block KT, Chandarana H, Kim S, Xu J, et al.

Golden-angle radial sparse parallel MRI: Combination of compressed sensing, parallel imaging, and golden-angle radial sampling for fast and flexible dynamic volumetric MRI. Magnetic Resonance in Medicine. 2014;**72**(3):707-717. DOI: 10.1002/mrm.24980

[75] Larkin S, Karavitaki N, Ansorge O. Rathke's cleft cyst. Handbook of Clinical Neurology. 2014;**124**:255-269. DOI: 10.1016/B978-0-444-59602-4.00017-4

[76] Wang S, Nie Q, Wu Z, Zhang J, Wei L. MRI and pathological features of Rathke cleft cysts in the sellar region. Experimental and Therapeutic Medicine. 2020;**19**(1):611-618. DOI: 10.3892/etm.2019.8272

[77] Muller HL, Merchant TE, Warmuth-Metz M, Martinez-Barbera JP, Puget S. Craniopharyngioma. Natural Review in Diseases Primers. 2019;**5**(1):75. DOI: 10.1038/s41572-019-0125-9

[78] Shikuma J, Kan K, Ito R, Hara K, Sakai H, Miwa T, et al. Critical review of IgG4-related hypophysitis. Pituitary. 2017;**20**(2):282-291. DOI: 10.1007/s11102-016-0773-7

[79] Iravani A, Osman MM, Weppler AM, Wallace R, Galligan A, Lasocki A, et al. FDG PET/CT for tumoral and systemic immune response monitoring of advanced melanoma during first-line combination ipilimumab and nivolumab treatment. European Journal of Nuclear Medicine and Molecular Imaging. 2020;**47**(12):2776-2786. DOI: 10.1007/s00259-020-04815-w

[80] Mekki A, Dercle L, Lichtenstein P, Nasser G, Marabelle A, Champiat S, et al. Machine learning defined diagnostic criteria for differentiating pituitary metastasis from autoimmune hypophysitis in patients undergoing immune checkpoint blockade therapy. European Journal of Cancer. 2019;**119**:44-56. DOI: 10.1016/j.ejca.2019.06.020

[81] Angelousi A, Cohen C, Sosa S, Danilowicz K, Papanastasiou L, Tsoli M, et al. Clinical, endocrine and imaging characteristics of patients with primary Hypophysitis. Hormone and Metabolic Research. 2018;**50**(4):296-302. DOI: 10.1055/s-0044-101036

[82] Lasocki A, Iravani A, Galligan A. The imaging of immunotherapy-related hypophysitis and other pituitary lesions in oncology patients. Clinical Radiology. 2021;**76**(5):325-332. DOI: 10.1016/j.crad.2020.12.028

[83] Tosaka M, Higuchi T, Horiguchi K, Osawa T, Arisaka Y, Fujita H, et al. Preoperative evaluation of Sellar and Parasellar macrolesions by [(18)F] Fluorodeoxyglucose positron emission tomography. World Neurosurgery. 2017;**103**:591-599. DOI: 10.1016/j.wneu.2017.04.032

Chapter 4

Characteristics of Magnetic Resonance Spectroscopy in Toxic Leukoencephalopathy

Zhiwei Zhou and Ping Xu

Abstract

Toxic leukoencephalopathy (TLE) refers to a series of diseases with central nervous system damage caused by poisoning of various toxic substances, including medications, gases, drugs, and ethanol as the main clinical manifestation. TLE mainly causes the damage to white matter fibers and subcortical gray matter nuclei, including basal ganglia nuclei, thalamus and brainstem nuclei (substantia nigra red nucleus), as well as cerebellar dentate nucleus, which manifests as altered mental status, epilepsy, paresthesia, hemiparesis, tetraparesis, or even death. Magnetic resonance spectroscopy (MRS) has contributed to understanding the etiology and stage of TLE. Moreover, the change of brain metabolites, which can be evaluated by MRS, provides additional information for confirming diagnosis, monitoring disease progression, and informing treatment response. In order to describe the MRS characteristics of TLE caused by different etiologies, we will review the spectroscopy change of TLE which is associated with psychoactive substances, immunosuppressant, chemotherapy, and environment (PICE). Therefore, we reviewed the MRS characteristics of heroin-induced TLE, methadone-induced TLE, oxycodone-induced TLE, Wernicke encephalopathy, Marchiafava-Bignami disease, methotrexate-related TLE, metronidazole-induced TLE, carbon monoxide-related encephalopathy, and toluene TLE in this chapter.

Keywords: magnetic resonance spectroscopy, psychoactive substances, immunosuppressant and chemotherapy, environment, leukoencephalopathy

1. Introduction

Toxic substances refer to the substances that enter the human body in small doses and can cause health damage through chemical or physical effects [1]. Poisoning refers to a kind of disease in which toxic substances enter the human body and cause biological function or structure change after reaching the toxic amount, resulting in temporary or permanent systemic damage [2]. When toxic substances damage the central nervous system, mainly causing white matter lesions, and some nerve nuclei and gray matter can also be affected, the occurrence of corresponding clinical manifestations is called toxic leukoencephalopathy (TLE) [3].

The neurotoxicology of toxic leukoencephalopathy has the following characteristics: (1) the degree of poisoning is positively correlated with the dose, duration, and concentration of toxin; (2) the cerebral lesions are generally symmetrical; (3) the initial symptoms of the disease are strongly related to the degree of poisoning; (4) the prognosis of patients with central nervous system involvement is unfavorable; and (5) toxic leukoencephalopathy can also have no obvious clinical symptoms.

MRI is the gold standard imaging modality to diagnose the diseases involving the white matter [4]. Magnetic resonance spectroscopy (MRS) is used to detect the change of brain metabolites in a specified region, which can provide additional information to establish diagnosis, differential diagnosis, monitor disease progression, and evaluate treatment response. MRS seems to be a new tool for understanding and diagnosing TLE.

2. Psychoactive substances-related TLE

Psychoactive substances refer to a series of chemical substances that can affect human mood, emotion, and behavior, change the state of consciousness, and have a dependency effect, also known as substances or addictive substances, including heroin, methadone, oxycodone, and alcohol, etc. Toxic leukoencephalopathy can be caused by abuse of psychoactive substances.

2.1 Heroin-induced TLE

Heroin has a strong dependence and toxic effects. Long-term abuse of heroin can cause systemic toxicity damage involving multiple systems and organs, such as brain, liver, heart, kidney and muscle damage, immune system, hematologic system, and reproductive system damage, among which brain damage is the most common. The damage to the central nervous system (CNS) caused by heroin inhalation or intravenous injection is commonly referred to as heroin-induced TLE. The reported CNS damage caused by heroin includes ischemic or hemorrhagic infarction, vasculitis, thrombosis, aneurysm, brain atrophy, and white matter cavernous degeneration. The main clinical symptoms are headache, memory loss, epilepsy, ataxia, paralysis, and other mental disorders [5–8].

Previous studies have described three clinical stages of heroin vapor-related leukoencephalopathy. The first stage is described as mostly cerebellar symptoms. And the second stage includes both cerebellar and extrapyramidal symptoms. Then the third stage progresses to spasms and akinetic mutism or hypotonic mutism [6]. These clinically recognized stages are related to the degree of white matter involvement on MRI.

MRI showed diffuse symmetric hypointense lesions involving the bilateral periventricular white matter, basal ganglia, brain stem, and superior cerebellum on T1-weighted images (T1WI) and fluid attenuated inversion recovery images (FLAIR), with hyperintensity on T2-weighted images (T2WI), without gadolinium enhancement, and sparing of the subcortical regions, and diffusion restriction on diffusion-weighted images (DWI) in the acute and subacute stages, nonrestricted diffusion appearances in chronic stage [6, 7]. However, some studies showed normal water diffusion on DWI and apparent diffusion coefficient (ADC) mapping in the acute stage. MRS showed increased lactate (Lac) and myo-inositol (mI), decreased N-acetyl aspartate (NAA) and creatine (Cr), normal to slightly decreased choline (Cho), and normal lipid peak in the affected white matter in acute stage. Repeated MRS in chronic stage showed persistent decrease of subcortical NAA/Cr ratio and mI, but partly improve, and significantly reduce of Cho/Cr ratio [6].

MRS revealed the Cho/Cr ratio was low in cortex but was normal in the cerebellum. The Lac/ Cr ratio in cerebellum was significantly increased in patients with the worst clinical condition. The Lac/Cr ratio in Cortex was only increased in the clinically worst patients and dramatically decreased in chronic stage with the corresponding clinical improvement [9]. A metabolic effect from a heroin-related toxin causing mitochondrial dysfunction was postulated.

2.2 Methadone-induced TLE

Methadone is a synthetic μ-opioid receptor agonist, with pharmacologic and analgesic properties similar to those of morphine, is usually used as a substitute therapy for drug abuse or dependence, and is also used to control intractable pain. Overdose of methadone, generally related to pain management, may lead to shallow breathing, unresponsive, pulseless, gait abnormalities, cognitive impairment, even respiratory depression resulting in anoxia, and followed by coma or death. Brain MRI was normal, or showed bilateral white matter hyperintense lesions on T2WI, and revealed extensive bilateral restricted-diffusion lesions throughout white matter on DWI, and hypointense on ADC in the acute stage [10].

In the subacute stage, MRI showed extensive and symmetric hyperintensity abnormalities in the deep white matter of both cerebral hemispheres on FLAIR and T2WI, with sparing of the subcortical U-fibers. And the affected areas had hyperintensity on diffusion-weighted trace images, but without corresponding diffusion restriction on ADC. MRS found a marked decrease of the NAA peak with a relative increase of the Cho peak and a Lac peak [11]. In the chronic stage, MRS showed reduced NAA and increased Cho levels in white matter, and relatively normal gray matter NAA/Cr ratios, with partial normalization of metabolites over time [10].

2.3 Oxycodone-induced TLE

Oxycodone-induced TLE presents as altered mental status and decreased respiratory effort, akathisia can also present with a biphasic clinical presentation of encephalopathy after oxycodone ingestion, and it occasionally leads to acute obstructive hydrocephalus [12]. The bilateral globi pallidi and cerebellar gray matter were preferentially affected, but cerebellar white matter and deep nuclei were spared. Oxycodone acts predominantly on μ-opioid receptors, which are located in the cerebellum and neostriatum, this localization is consistent with the areas of injury of patients on neuroimaging and argues that the opioids themselves are the toxic agent [12]. Opioid toxicity and genetic predisposition were proposed as possible pathogenesis.

Findings of brain MRI in the delayed leukoencephalopathy episode revealed hyperintense lesions in the bilateral globi pallidi, superficial cerebellar hemispheres, corpus callosum, bilateral cerebral peduncles, posterior limbs of the internal capsule, and right frontal subcortical white matter and multifocal punctate areas of multiple white matter tracts on T2WI and FLAIR, with associated contrast enhancement on T1WI, and with corresponding hyperintensity on T1WI, with punctate areas of diffusion restriction in white matter tracts on DWI, and hyperintensity in the bilateral cerebral hemispheres on T2WI and FLAIR with sparing of the cerebellar white matter and deep cerebellar nuclei, are consistent with a subacute toxic encephalopathy related to oxycodone intoxication. MRS in delayed toxic leukoencephalopathy has demonstrated decreased NAA and Cho peaks with an elevated lactate peak in affected white matter in the acute stage. MRS showed qualitatively decreased NAA, Cho, and

Cr peaks in the globi pallidi, with normal metabolite ratios, without significant lactate peak in the subacute stage, which supports the diagnosis of a subacute opioid toxic encephalopathy given the decreased metabolite peaks without a Lac peak [12].

2.4 Wernicke encephalopathy

Wernicke encephalopathy is a metabolic disease of the CNS caused by vitamin B1 deficiency, which partly develops in patients with alcohol abuse [13]. Only 1/3 of the patients showed the classic triad of manifestations, namely, ophthalmoplegia, ataxia, and altered mental status. Most of the patients were complicated in the late stage of various related diseases, and the symptoms of different diseases were intertwined and coexisted.

The typical MRI findings of Wernicke encephalopathy patients are bilateral and symmetrical hyperintense lesions in the mammillary bodies, thalami, tectal plate, and periaqueductal area on T2WI and FLAIR [14]. A previous MRS study found that the NAA/Cr ratio decreased in the thalami and cerebellum and a lactate peak in the cerebellum in the acute stage, and the NAA/Cr ratio increased in the thalami after thiamine supplement, but NAA/Cr ratio did not improve in the cerebellum in the chronic stage. Another research revealed a decreased NAA/Cr ratio without detectable lactate in the thalami in the subacute stage, and NAA/Cr ratio increased after thiamine administration. However, the other research reported that a remarkable increased lactate level in the thalami, but without NAA/Cr ratio changes in the acute stage [14–16].

2.5 Marchiafava-Bignami disease

Marchiafava-Bignami disease (MBD) is a rare disease associated with alcoholism, the prevalence of which is less than 0.002% in alcoholics [17]. The pathological characteristics are symmetrical demyelination, necrosis, and atrophy of the corpus callosum, extra-callosal white matter can be simultaneously affected, even the cortex [18]. The clinical manifestations of MBD lack specificity, which manifested as unconsciousness, confusion, delirium, mutism, seizures, and brain disconnection syndrome [19]. In the era where the diagnosis depended on the pathological manifestations at autopsy, MBD was considered a fatal disease [20]. The accuracy and number of antemortem diagnoses were greatly improved after the extensive application of neuroimaging techniques [19]. However, only a few patients achieved favorable recovery after treatment, and most had poor outcomes.

MRI plays an important role in the diagnosis of MBD. In the acute stage, symmetrical lesions in the corpus callosum with hypointensity or isointensity on T1WI and hyperintensity on T2WI and FLAIR, without obvious mass effect, and the lesions can extend to the adjacent white matter [21–23]. DWI showed hyperintensity in the lesions, with hypointensity on ADC [24]. Some patients with gadolinium-enhanced in lesions in the corpus callosum [25]. With the progression of the disease to the subacute and chronic stage, necrosis and cystic degeneration can appear in the corpus callosum, with hypointensity on T1WI and hypointensity on T2WI and FLAIR in the center part of the lesions, and hyperintensity in the peripheral part of the lesions, especially in the genu and splenium of corpus callosum [26]. DWI showed restricted diffusion in the center part of the lesions of the corpus callosum, and with restricted diffusion in the peripheral part [25]. Moreover, no abnormal contrast enhancement was observed, and the corpus callosum atrophied and thinned, and was particularly clear and intuitive on sagittal scans [25].

In previous studies, MRS was usually performed in the acute phase of MBD, the corpus callosum was the most commonly selected region of interest, followed by periventricular white matter and right parietal region, occasionally in anterior central gyrus [27–34]. In the acute phase, MRS showed that decreased NAA peak and NAA/Cr ratio, a slightly increased Cho peak and Cho/Cr ratio, and a Lac peak could be observed [27–29, 31, 32, 34]. In the subacute phase, there is a decrease in NAA/Cr ratio, a partial and gradual decrease in Cho/Cr ratio, and a Lac peak in some patients were observed [30, 31, 33]. In the chronic phase, the NAA/Cr ratio partially recovered and the Cho/Cr ratio gradually decreased. The temporary dysfunction of axons can explain the partial recovery of NAA/Cr ratio, and the decrease of Cho/Cr ratio is synchronized with the chronic phase of demyelinating. Lac was initially replaced by lipid peak in chronic phase, which was consistent with axonal injury [30, 35]. Lac or lipid peaks were not obvious after nearly 1 year of symptoms. MRS findings suggested that metabolites change over time and supported the pathogenic theory that inflammatory response may be accompanied by MBD demyelination and micronecrosis. The resonance signals of taurine and scyllo inositol increased significantly when observing the brain of MBD patients who abstained from alcohol by MRS [30].

3. Immunosuppressant-related TLE

3.1 Methotrexate-related TLE

Methotrexate is an anticancer and immunomodulatory drug. Methotrexate-related TLE is a rare complication in methotrexate therapy. The severity of methotrexate-related TLE ranges from mild reversible leukoencephalopathy to irreversible and even fatal disseminated necrotizing leukoencephalopathy. Methotrexate-related TLE can occur even with low-dose administration and can especially develop with intrathecal or intravenous administration. The most frequently reported symptom was seizures, followed by nonspecific symptoms such as cognitive dysfunction, disorientation, headaches, and visual disturbances [36].

The typical MRI findings are symmetrical hyperintense lesions in white matter, brainstem, basal ganglia, thalamus, cerebellum, and even spinal cord on T2WI and FLAIR, with restricted diffusion on DWI and on ADC, with or without gadolinium enhancement. The limited published data from MRS studies showed a reduced NAA and Cr and an elevated Cho with or without a lactate peak, which may be associated with an acute demyelinating mechanism [36].

3.2 Metronidazole-related TLE

Metronidazole is widely used in a variety of infectious conditions and with good tolerance and has been used to help diminish or control the signs and symptoms of inflammatory bowel disease, its adverse reactions rarely occur in peripheral neuritis and brain damage, which are mostly transient and reversible, but few persistent nerve damage [37]. MRI findings of an adolescent patient with Down syndrome and Crohn's disease treated with metronidazole revealed hyperintense lesions in the corpus callosum, basal ganglia, brainstem, substantia nigra pars compacta, red nucleus, globus pallidus, putamen, caudate, and cerebellum on T2WI and FLAIR, with slightly contrast enhancement of the lesions in the red nucleus and cerebral peduncles. MRS examination demonstrated a persistent Lac elevation during metronidazole treatment in the splenium and basal ganglia. Repeat MRI and spectroscopy studies showed new lesions in the medial thalami and a persistent lactate resonance in addition to the previously described abnormalities. Repeat MRI at 3 months follow-up showed near-complete resolution of the previous abnormalities, MRS shows resolution of elevated lactate peak, lower spectral signal-to-noise ratio reflects reduced volume sampled within the splenium [37]. The findings on MRS suggest the possibility of a reversible mitochondrial dysfunction as a cause of the abnormalities.

4. Chemotherapy-related TLE

4.1 Methotrexate-induced leukoencephalopathy

Methotrexate is a commonly used antimetabolic drug, which is widely used in the treatment of leukemia, lymphoma, and osteosarcoma. Methotrexate interferes with DNA synthesis by inhibiting dihydrofolate reductase, an enzyme that plays a crucial role in reducing folate, which plays an important role in DNA synthesis. The incidence of MTX-induced leukoencephalopathy ranges from 3–10%. Studies reported the restricted diffusion on DWI, which is an early sign to accurately diagnose acute MTX-induced leukoencephalopathy [38]. The brain MRI showed widespread periventricular hyperintensity on FLAIR, and with a specific pattern of restricted diffusion on DWI, MRS showed a slight elevation of the Cho peak with a normal NAA/Cho ratio, indicating multifocal supratentorial neuronal losses suggested a demyelinating process, which was more consistent with leukoencephalopathy [38].

5. Environment-related TLE

5.1 Carbon monoxide-related encephalopathy

Delayed encephalopathy due to carbon monoxide intoxication refers to the patients with acute carbon monoxide (CO) poisoning at first, then suddenly developed series of nervous system manifestations, mainly including dementia, altered mental state, pyramidal and extrapyramidal symptoms, and even coma after complete clinical recovery, the duration is usually ranging from 2 to 40 days.

Diagnosis was based on present history of exposure to CO, blood carboxyhemoglobin concentration in arterial blood immediately after admission and presence of acute neurological symptoms on admission, and series of nervous system manifestations after a lucid interval. Acute low-dose CO intoxication seems to cause reversible neuropsychological impairment whereas patients' exposure to high-dose CO may show a complex clinical pattern, that is, delayed encephalopathy and neuropsychiatric sequelae may occur after a lucid interval of 3 days to 4 weeks after the initial recovery from the acute stage. Although neuropsychiatric disorders are common, delayed encephalopathy is a rare and unclear complication.

MRI is routinely used to illustrate abnormalities in the CO-intoxicated brain. Cerebral MRI showed symmetrical and diffuse hypointensity on lesions in the centrum semiovale and periventricular white matter on T1WI, with hyperintensity on T2WI and DWI, and mild hypointensity or isointensity on ADC in the ultra-acute or acute phase. All of these hyperintense lesions on T2WI and DWI with low ADC in the CWM persisted in the subacute and chronic phases. In severe cases, the lesions could also appear in the subcortical white matter, corpus callosum, and internal and external capsules. Additionally, the pathognomonic sign of CO intoxication is the lesions in the globus pallidus [39].

MRS studies demonstrated increased Cho peak and Cho/Cr ratio and reduced NAA peak and NAA/Cr ratio in the white matter, gray matter, and basal ganglia in the early period, and a Lac peak appeared in subacute stage, with an increased Lac/Cr ratio [39–45]. The persistent increase of Cho was thought to reflect the course of progressive demyelination. The appearance of lactate and decrease in NAA reflected that the neuron injury became irreversible. Patients with Lac peak persisted after the NAA and Cho peaks had disappeared in the chronic stage were supposed to show poor prognoses, because extensive neuronal tissue is irreversibly damaged. After starting hyperbaric oxygen therapy, the Cho/Cr ratio in the white matter started to decrease and the lactate peak disappeared in chronic stage [45]. The NAA/Cr ratio gradually increased and did not return to the normal range. MRS showed metabolites in the gray matter had reverted to normal in chronic stage, consistent with neuronal recovery [39]. In white matter and centrum semiovale, NAA/Cr had almost returned to normal, Lac was no longer significantly detected, and mI/Cr had further increased, consistent with chronic gliosis [41–43].

Compared with patients with transit acute symptoms only, the mean Cho/Cr ratios in bilateral centrum semiovale were significantly higher in patients with delayed neuropsychiatric sequelae, and no significant difference in mean NAA/Cr ratio between the above two groups [41]. These findings suggest that the Cho/Cr ratio in the subacute phase after CO intoxication represents inflammation accompanied by demyelination in the centrum semiovale, and can predict chronic neurological symptoms [41].

5.2 Toluene TLE

Toluene, which is an organic solvent, inhaling of a large amount of toluene mainly causes inhibition of central nervous system. The myelin sheath structure of the central nervous system is rich in lipids. Toluene can easily enter the lipid-rich brain parenchyma through the blood-brain barrier, and damage the cell membrane, resulting in pathological and physiological changes such as nerve tissue demyelination, gliosis, and iron deposition, thus causing a series of clinical manifestations such as toxic brain disease. Toluene TLE is caused by long-term inhalation of toluene, characterized by cognitive impairment, headache, blurred vision, insomnia, hands tremors, and ataxia. These clinical manifestations lack specificity. MRI showed diffuse and symmetric hyperintense lesions in subcortical white matter, deep white matter, bilateral external capsule, bilateral globus pallidus, bilateral thalamus, and bilateral cerebellar dentate nuclei on T2WI and FLAIR, with hypointensity on T1WI, restricted diffusion in the same regions on DWI, and reduced ADC value. The most characteristic feature is the symmetrical "bracket" shaped hyperintense lesions of the bilateral external capsules on T2WI. ASL showed normal CBF in the bilateral white matter, cortical gray matter, and basal ganglia. MRS revealed that decreased NAA peak and increased Cho peak, decreased NAA/Cr ratio, and increased Cho/Cr ratio in the corona radiata [46].

Compared with the health control, the NAA/Cr ratio in the cerebellum and centrum semiovale of the toluene abusers was significantly lower, but mI/Cr was higher. Furthermore, no significant difference was found in the NAA/Cr, Cho/Cr, and mI/Cr ratios of the thalami. There was no difference Cho/Cr ratios between toluene abusers and control group. The NAA/Cr and mI/Cr ratios in cerebellum and centrum semiovale were significantly associated with the duration of abuse [47].

6. Conclusion

The clinical manifestations of patients with TLE are often lack of specificity. TLE is usually related to psychoactive substances, immunosuppressant, chemotherapy, and environment (PICE), and the diagnosis is based on a history of exposure to toxic substances, clinical symptoms and signs, corresponding toxic substances found in laboratory tests, MRI suggests symmetrical white matter damage, with or without deep brain nuclei and cerebellar lesions. Meanwhile, MRS can reveal the changes of metabolites in the affected lesions at different stages, as a supplementary means of clinical and conventional neuroimaging. Therefore, MRS is helpful for the diagnosis and differential diagnosis of TLE and can provide information on metabolic abnormalities of early lesions.

Conflict of interest

The authors declare no conflict of interest.

Notes/thanks/other declarations

None.

Acronyms and abbreviations

TLE	Toxic leukoencephalopathy
MRS	Magnetic resonance spectroscopy
CNS	the central nervous system
T1WI	T1-weighted images
FLAIR	fluid attenuated inversion recovery images
T2WI	T2-weighted images
DWI	diffusion-weighted images
ADC	apparent diffusion coefficient
Lac	lactate
mI	myo-inositol
NAA	N-acetyl aspartate
Cr	creatine
Cho	choline
MBD	Marchiafava-Bignami disease
CO	carbon monoxide

Author details

Zhiwei Zhou and Ping Xu*
Department of Neurology, Affiliated Hospital of Zunyi Medical University, Zunyi, China

*Address all correspondence to: xuping527@vip.sina.com

References

[1] Harbord N. Poisoning, toxicology, and the nephrologist. Advances in Chronic Kidney Disease. 2020;**27**:3-4. DOI: 10.1053/j.ackd.2019.10.002

[2] Zhang Y, Yu B, Wang N, et al. Acute poisoning in Shenyang, China: A retrospective and descriptive study from 2012 to 2016. BMJ Open. 2018;**8**:e021881. DOI: 10.1136/bmjopen-2018-021881

[3] Assaf R, Michael PG, Langford N. Nitrous oxide-induced toxic leukoencephalopathy. BMJ Case Reports. 2020;**13**:e238315. DOI: 10.1136/bcr-2020-238315

[4] Beitinjaneh A, McKinney AM, Cao Q, et al. Toxic leukoencephalopathy following fludarabine-associated hematopoietic cell transplantation. Biology of Blood and Marrow Transplantation. 2011;**17**:300-308. DOI: 10.1016/j.bbmt.2010.04.003

[5] Hedley-Whyte ET. Leukoence phalopathy and raised brain lactate from heroin vapor inhalation. Neurology. 2000;**54**:2027-2028. DOI: 10.1212/wnl.54.10.2027-b

[6] Kashyap S, Majeed G, Bowen I, et al. Toxic leukoencephalopathy due to inhalational heroin abuse. Annals of Indian Academy of Neurology. 2020;**23**:542-544. DOI: 10.4103/aian.AIAN_446_18

[7] Offiah C, Hall E. Heroin-induced leukoencephalopathy: Characterization using MRI, diffusion-weighted imaging, and MR spectroscopy. Clinical Radiology. 2008;**63**:146-152. DOI: 10.1016/j.crad.2007.07.021

[8] Jee RC, Tsao WL, Shyu WC, et al. Heroin vapor inhalation-induced spongiform leukoencephalopathy. Journal of the Formosan Medical Association. 2009;**108**:518-522. DOI: 10.1016/S0929-6646(09)60101-7

[9] Bartlett E, Mikulis DJ. Chasing "chasing the dragon" with MRI: Leukoencephalopathy in drug abuse. British Journal of Radiology. 2005;**78**:997-1004. DOI: 10.1259/bjr/61535842

[10] Huisa BN, Gasparovic C, Taheri S, et al. Imaging of subacute blood-brain barrier disruption after methadone overdose. Journal of Neuroimaging. 2013;**23**:441-444. DOI: 10.1111/j.1552-6569.2011.00669.x

[11] Salgado RA, Jorens PG, Baar I, et al. Methadone-induced toxic leukoencephalopathy: MR imaging and MR proton spectroscopy findings. AJNR: American Journal of Neuroradiology. 2010;**31**:565-566. DOI: 10.3174/ajnr.A1889

[12] Beatty CW, Ko PR, Nixon J, et al. Delayed-onset movement disorder and encephalopathy after oxycodone ingestion. Seminars in Pediatric Neurology. 2014;**21**:160-165. DOI: 10.1016/j.spen.2014.06.009

[13] Kim TE, Lee EJ, Young JB, et al. Wernicke encephalopathy and ethanol-related syndromes. Seminars in Ultrasound Ct and Mri. 2014;**35**:85-96. DOI: 10.1053/j.sult.2013.09.004

[14] Manzo G, De Gennaro A, Cozzolino A, et al. MR imaging findings in alcoholic and nonalcoholic acute Wernicke's encephalopathy: A review. Biomed Research International. 2014;**2014**:503596. DOI: 10.1155/2014/503596

[15] Murata T, Fujito T, Kimura H, et al. Serial MRI and 1 H-MRS of Wernicke's encephalopathy: Report of a case with remarkable cerebellar lesions on MRI. Psychiatry Research. 2001;**108**:49-55. DOI: 10.1016/s0925-4927(01)00304-3

[16] Mascalchi M, Belli G, Guerrini L, et al. Proton MR spectroscopy of Wernicke encephalopathy. AJNR: American Journal of Neuroradiology. 2002;**23**:1803-1806

[17] Zahr NM, Pfefferbaum A. Alcohol's effects on the brain: Neuroimaging results in humans and animal models. Alcohol Research: Current Reviews. 2017;**38**:183-206

[18] Sato Y, Tabira T, Tateishi J. Marchiafava-Bignami disease, striatal degeneration, and other neurological complications of chronic alcoholism in a Japanese. Acta Neuropathologica. 1981;**53**:15-20. DOI: 10.1007/bf00697179

[19] Hillbom M, Saloheimo P, Fujioka S, et al. Diagnosis and management of Marchiafava-Bignami disease: A review of CT/MRI confirmed cases. Journal of Neurology Neurosurgery and Psychiatry. 2014;**85**:168-173. DOI: 10.1136/jnnp-2013-305979

[20] Ironside R, Bosanquet FD, McMenemey WH. Central demyelination of the corpus callosum (Marchiafava-Bignami disease) with report of a second case in Great Britain. Brain. 1961;**84**: 212-230. DOI: 10.1093/brain/84.2.212

[21] Zhou Z, Li Q, Zeng L, et al. Marchiafava-Bignami disease concurrent with intracerebral hemorrhage: A case description. Quantitative Imaging in Medicine and Surgery. 2022;**12**: 2596-2601. DOI: 10.21037/qims-21-901

[22] Xu T, Guo K. A rare MRI finding in a patient with Marchiafava-Bignami disease. Neurological Sciences. 2021;**42**:5419-5420. DOI: 10.1007/s10072-021-05685-2

[23] Tiwari S, Dubey P, Swami MK, et al. Classical imaging finding in Marchiafava Bignami disease. Neurology India. 2021;**69**:1627-1628. DOI: 10.4103/0028-3886.333487

[24] Renard D, Le Goff JM, Guillamo JS, et al. Reversible "ears of the lynx" sign in Marchiafava-Bignami disease. Acta Neurologica Belgica. 2019;**119**:275-277. DOI: 10.1007/s13760-018-0989-6

[25] Wang Z, Wang J, Yi F, et al. Gadolinium enhancement may indicate a condition at risk of developing necrosis in Marchiafava-Bignami disease: A case report and literature review. Frontiers in Human Neuroscience. 2019;**13**:79. DOI: 10.3389/fnhum.2019.00079

[26] Lakatos A, Kosta P, Konitsiotis S, et al. Marchiafava-Bignami disease: An acquired callosotomy. Neurology. 2014;**83**:1219. DOI: 10.1212/wnl.0000000000000811

[27] Quintas-Neves M, Amorim JM, Soares-Fernandes JP. Marchiafava-Bignami disease: Two chronologically distinct stages in the same patient. Canadian Journal of Neurological Sciences. 2020;**47**:689-690. DOI: 10.1017/cjn.2020.86

[28] Nalini A, Kovoor JME, Dawn R, et al. Marchiafava-Bignami disease: Two cases with magnetic resonance imaging and positron emission tomography scan findings. Neurology India. 2009;**57**: 644-648. DOI: 10.4103/0028-3886.57813

[29] Tuntiyatorn L, Laothamatas J. Acute Marchiafava-Bignami disease with callosal, cortical, and white matter involvement. Emergency Radiology. 2008;**15**:137-140. DOI: 10.1007/s10140-007-0640-y

[30] Gambini A, Falini A, Moiola L, et al. Marchiafava-Bignami disease: Longitudinal MR imaging and MR spectroscopy study. AJNR: American Journal of Neuroradiology. 2003;**24**:249-253

[31] Lee SH, Kim SS, Kim SH, et al. Acute Marchiafava-Bignami disease with selective involvement of the precentral cortex and splenium a serial magnetic resonance imaging study. Neurologist. 2011;**17**:213-217. DOI: 10.1097/NRL.0b013e31821a25ae

[32] Consoli A, Pirritano D, Bosco D, et al. Corticosteroid treatment in a patient with Marchiafava-Bignami disease. Neurological Sciences. 2014;**35**:1143-1145. DOI: 10.1007/s10072-014-1705-9

[33] Sarpa MG, Ferrazzoli D, Massa R, et al. Paucisymptomatic Marchiafava-Bignami disease with relevant diffusion-weighted MRI lesions. International Journal of Neuroscience. 2013;**123**:738-740. DOI: 10.3109/00207454.2013.795150

[34] Machado A, Soares-Fernandes J, Ribeiro M, et al. Alcohol abuse and acute behavioural disturbances in a 24-year-old patient. Journal of Clinical Neuroscience. 2009;**16**:811. DOI: 10.1016/j.jocn.2008.08.040

[35] Zhou Z, Li Q, Pan C, et al. Magnetic resonance spectroscopy and gadolinium enhancement assist in the diagnosis of nonalcoholic Marchiafava-Bignami disease with necrosis lesions: A case description. Quantitative Imaging in Medicine and Surgery. 2022;**12**:1652-1657. DOI: 10.21037/qims-21-632

[36] Gonzalez-Suarez I, Aguilar-Amat MJ, Trigueros M, et al. Leukoencephalopathy due to oral methotrexate. Cerebellum. 2014;**13**:178-183. DOI: 10.1007/s12311-013-0528-1

[37] Cecil K, Halsted MJ, Schapiro M, et al. Reversible MR imaging and MR spectroscopy abnormalities in association with metronidazole therapycecil. Journal of Computer Assisted Tomography. 2002;**26**:948-951. DOI: 10.1097/00004728-200211000-00016

[38] Doan N, Patel M, Nguyen HS, et al. Methotrexate-induced leukoencephalopathy without typical restricted diffusion on diffusion-weighted imaging and the utility of magnetic resonance spectroscopy to support the diagnosis. Asian Journal of Neurosurgery. 2018;**13**:848-850. DOI: 10.4103/ajns.AJNS_324_16

[39] Hansen MB, Kondziella D, Danielsen ER, et al. Cerebral proton magnetic resonance spectroscopy demonstrates reversibility of N-acetylaspartate/creatine in gray matter after delayed encephalopathy due to carbon monoxide intoxication: A case report. Journal of Medical Case Reports. 2014;**8**:211. DOI: 10.1186/1752-1947-8-211

[40] Sakamoto K, Murata T, Omori M, et al. Clinical studies on three cases of the interval form of carbon monoxide poisoning: Serial proton magnetic resonance spectroscopy as a prognostic predictor. Psychiatry Research. 1998;**83**:179-192. DOI: 0.1016/s0925-4927(98)00038-9

[41] Beppu T, Nishimoto H, Fujiwara S, et al. 1H-magnetic resonance spectroscopy indicates damage to cerebral white matter in the subacute phase after CO poisoning. Journal of Neurology Neurosurgery and Psychiatry. 2011;**82**:869-875. DOI: 10.1136/jnnp.2010.222422

[42] Robin A, Hurley R, et al. Applications of functional imaging to carbon monoxide poisoning. Journal of Neuropsychiatry and Clinical

Neurosciences. 2001;**13**:157-160. DOI: 10.1176/jnp.13.2.157

[43] Murata T, Itoh S, Koshino T, et al. Serial proton magnetic resonance spectroscopy in a patient with the interval form of carbon monoxide poisoning. Journal of Neurology Neurosurgery and Psychiatry. 1995;**58**:100-103. DOI: 10.1136/jnnp.58.1.100

[44] Prockop LD. Carbon monoxide brain toxicity: Clinical, magnetic resonance imaging, magnetic resonance spectroscopy, and neuropsychological effects in 9 people. Journal of Neuroimaging. 2005;**15**:144-149. DOI: 10.1177/1051228404273819

[45] Terajima K, Igarashi H, Hirose M, et al. Serial assessments of delayed encephalopathy after carbon monoxide poisoning using magnetic resonance spectroscopy and diffusion tensor imaging on 3.0T system. European Neurology. 2008;**59**:55-61. DOI: 10.1159/000109262

[46] Fan Z, Luo F, Wang Q, et al. Preliminary study on proton MR spectroscopy of DNS. Chinese Journal of Medical Imaging Technology. 2008;**24**:1708-1710

[47] Aydin K, Sencer S, Ogel K, et al. Single-voxel proton MR spectroscopy in toluene abuse. Magnetic Resonance Imaging. 2003;**21**:777-785. DOI: 10.1016/s0730-725x(03)00175-9

Chapter 5

Neuroimaging in Neonates: Newer Insights

Manikandasamy Veluchamy

Abstract

Neuroimaging plays a key role in management of critically ill neonates with neurological problems. Magnetic Resonance Imaging (MRI) is the most commonly used neuroimaging modality in evaluation of neonatal encephalopathy, because MRI provides better image quality and accurate delineation of the lesion. Newer modalities of MRI like Diffusion Weighted Imaging (DWI), Diffusion Tensor Imaging (DTI) are useful in identifying the brain lesion and also in predicting the neurodevelopmental outcome. Magnetic Resonance Angiography (MRA) and Magnetic Resonance Venography (MRV) are used to assess the cerebral arteries and veins with or without the use of contrast material. Arterial Spin Labelling (ASL) MRI and Phase Contrast (PC) MRI are newer modalities of MRI used to assess the cerebral perfusion without the use of contrast material. Magnetic Resonance Spectroscopy (MRS) is a functional MRI modality used to assess the level of brain metabolites which help us in diagnosing neuro metabolic disorders, peroxisomal disorders and mitochondrial disorders. Several predictive scores are available based on the size and location of lesions in MRI, and these scores are used to predict the neurodevelopmental outcome in term neonates with encephalopathy. MRI at term equivalent age in preterm neonates used to predict neurodevelopmental outcome in later life.

Keywords: neuroimaging, magnetic resonance imaging, diffusion weighted imaging, diffusion tensor imaging, magnetic resonance spectroscopy, arterial spin labelling

1. Introduction

Neuroimaging is an important and inevitable modality in diagnosis of critically ill neonates with neurological problems, and also helps in prognostication. Currently cranial ultrasonography (CUS), computerised tomography (CT), and magnetic resonance imaging (MRI) are the most widely available neuroimaging modalities for the evaluation of critically ill neonates. The ideal neuroimaging technique gives us information which helps in identifying the underlying diagnosis, determine the management and in predicting the neurodevelopmental outcome.

2. Cranial ultrasonography

CUS still remains the most popular neuroimaging modality, even though advanced neuroimaging techniques like CT and MRI are available. The presence of fontanelles in neonates provides an acoustic window for neuroimaging using CUS.

The main advantages of CUS are that it can be done at bedside, absence of ionising radiation, can be repeated many times and there is no need for sedation. Even though CUS can be used to detect congenital anomalies of brain, congenital infections and in identification of hemorrhagic, ischemic and cystic lesions of brain, now a days CUS is mainly used in screening all preterm neonates born before 32 weeks for clinically unsuspected Intraventricular Hemorrhage (IVH), Peri Ventricular Leukomalacia (PVL), and Ventriculomegaly due to Post Hemorrhagic Hydrocephalus [1].

The role of CUS in term neonates is very less in this current era. In neonates with hypoxic ischemic encephalopathy, abnormalities in cerebral blood flow may be the early sign which can be diagnosed with transcranial doppler ultrasound, but the role of CUS as sole imaging modality in term neonates with encephalopathy is very limited. CUS can be used as a initial screening modality followed by MRI as definitive neuroimaging modality.

The main limitation of CUS in neonates is the posterior fossa could not be visualized properly, and subtle anomalies in the grey white matter can be missed due to lack of myelination in the neonatal brain.

3. Computerised tomography

CT scan is very rarely used now as a neuroimaging technique in neonates because of the risk of exposure to harmful ionizing radiation and also the advent of safer MRI technique. In the past decade CT scan was considered more sensitive in detecting acute hemorrhage and calcifications in brain, which is replaced with the advent of advanced MR sequences with better image quality and higher field strength which delineates the calcifications and acute hemorrhage better. The main problem related to MRI is the longer scan times and the requirement of MRI compatible life support systems while scanning the critically ill neonate.

A comparative study between CT scan, conventional MRI and diffusion weighted MRI done in term newborns with encephalopathy showed Diffusion weighted MRI is the most sensitive technique in assessing brain injury in neonates with encephalopathy, especially for cortical injury, white matter injury and focal lesions such as stroke [2].

CT scan can be used as imaging modality in urgent situations when MRI is not available, and when baby's condition is too critically ill which will not allow longer scan times with MRI.

4. Magnetic resonance imaging

MRI is the most commonly used modality of neuroimaging in evaluation of Neonatal Encephalopathy. MRI is considered as the standard neuroimaging modality in term neonates with encephalopathy. Even though conventional MRI sequences are helpful in diagnosis of neurological problems, advanced MRI techniques such as Magnetic Resonance Spectroscopy (MRS) and Diffusion Weighted Imaging (DWI) are useful in identifying the exact etiology.

5. Indications for MRI in neonates

5.1 To identify the cause for neonatal encephalopathy

Neuroimaging plays a key role in diagnosis of genetic and metabolic disorders and it helps to differentiate metabolic disorders from other causes of neonatal encephalopathy (**Figure 1**) [3].

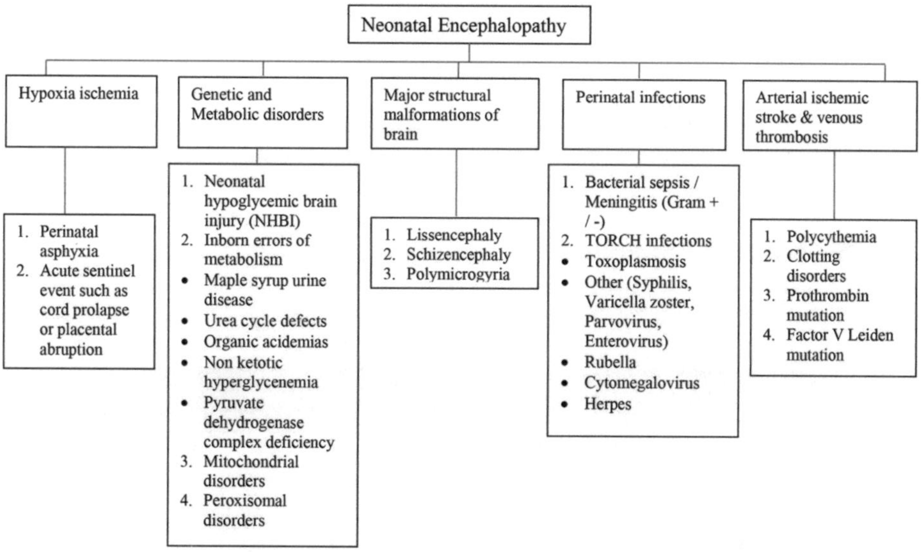

Figure 1.
Etiologies of neonatal encephalopathy.

5.2 To predict the neurodevelopmental outcome in Term neonates with HIE and in Very preterm neonates

6. Newer MRI techniques

Several newer MRI techniques are used now, which helps in enhancing the accuracy of diagnosis and also in prognostication.

6.1 Diffusion weighted imaging

DWI is currently an indispensable modality of neuroimaging. DWI having been used most commonly in adults for evaluation of stroke, currently it has been widely used in neonatal neuroimaging for both diagnosis and prognostic purposes.

DWI uses the diffusion properties of hydrogen molecules within the substance, when these hydrogen molecules move freely they diffuse away, so signal loss will occur in DWI. The movement of hydrogen molecules during application of magnetic gradient affects the signal and direction of movement of hydrogen molecules. When there is diffusion restriction or reduced diffusion, the movement of hydrogen molecules are limited which is seen as high signal intensity in DWI.

The quantitative calculation of diffusion or the rate of diffusion is expressed as the Apparent Diffusion Coefficient (ADC). ADC mapping used to find out the site and extent of injury. The areas with diffusion restriction appear brighter with high signal intensity in DWI and appear darker with low signal intensity in ADC mapping. ADC values should be interpreted cautiously after 1–2 weeks, because pseudonormalization occurs during the sub-acute stage after ischemic event had occurred. ADC pseudonormalization represents apparent return to normal values on ADC maps, but DWI still shows high signal intensity. This ADC pseudonormalization does not represent resolution of ischemic brain damage.

After an acute ischemic event, there is net shift of water from the fast diffusing extracellular compartment to slow diffusing intracellular compartment, hence there is a net slowing of water diffusion or diffusion restriction. In the sub-acute stage after an ischemic event, the cell walls break down in the infarcted area and there is increased diffusion. This increased diffusion in damaged tissues during the sub-acute stage is called pseudonormalization as the damaged tissues have diffusion equivalent to that of normal brain tissue. This pseudonormalization occurs after 2 weeks in myelinated brain but it occurs earlier in unmyelinated neonatal brain [4].

DWI can be used as supplemental MRI technique along with conventional MRI in recognising the pattern of brain damage and also in predicting the motor outcome [5].

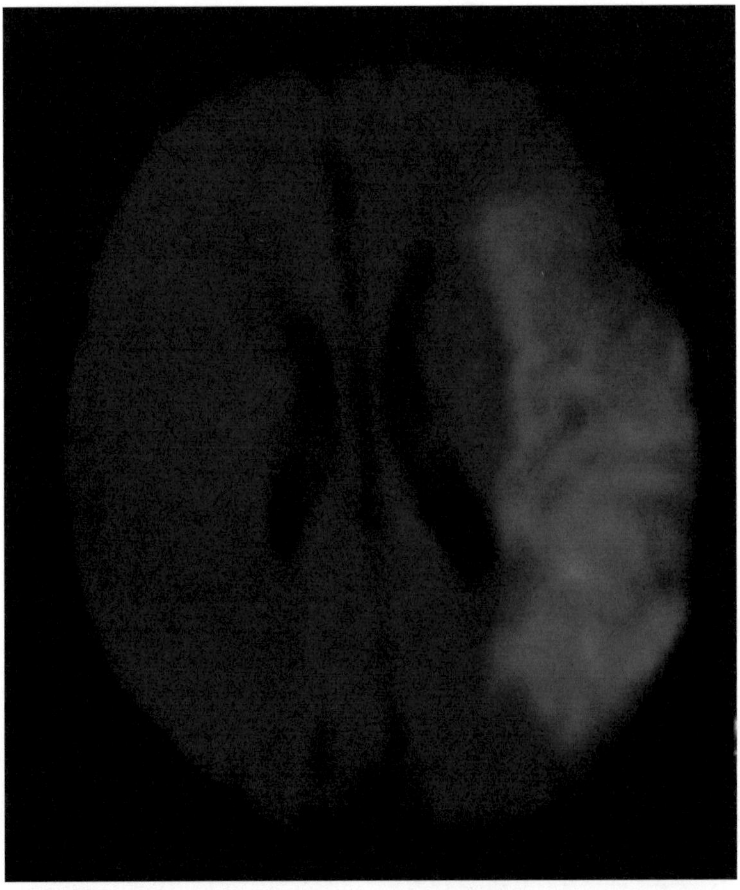

Figure 2.
Perinatal stroke DWI.

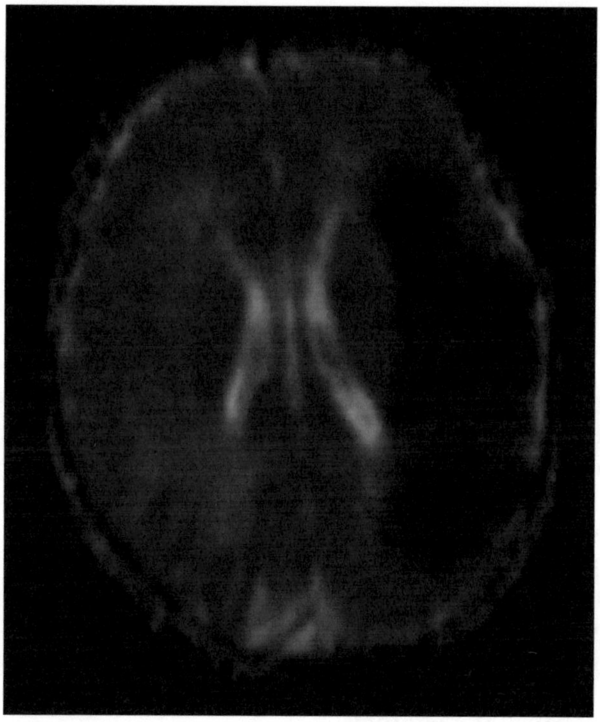

Figure 3.
Perinatal stroke ADC.

The below figures are the DWI and corresponding ADC mapping images of the neonate with stroke showing hyperintense lesions in DWI in the left temporo-parietal cortex and hypointense in ADC on the same location in brain (**Figures 2** and **3**).

DWI provides evidence of cerebral injury before conventional MRI in term babies with neonatal encephalopathy.

6.2 Diffusion tensor imaging

Diffusion Tensor Imaging (DTI) uses the property of diffusion anisotropy. The ADC of intracellular water is lower than that of extracellular water, because the movement of intracellular water is restricted by the intracellular structures and cell membrane. Myelin also impairs the exchange of water molecules across cell membranes. When water moves parallel to axons, it moves freely within the myelin layers without crossing the lipid membranes. The water ADC values are greater when parallel to axons than perpendicular to them. This spatial variation in ADC values within the brain is called diffusion anisotropy.

The diffusion anisotropy is evaluated and expressed as Fractional Anisotropy (FA) mapping. FA values usually ranging between 0 and 1. The anisotropy value of the white matter of neonatal brain is initially low and increases as the myelination increases.

The differences in regional diffusion of the brain structure used to study the myelination of brain as well as ischemic and non-ischemic areas of the brain.

In DWI magnetic resonance gradients are applied in one to three directions, but in Diffusion Tensor Imaging (DTI) magnetic resonance gradients are applied in many directions, from 6 to 30 or more.

Fractional anisotropy measured using DTI in full term neonates found that there is significant correlation between white matter structural variation and neurodevelopmental outcome [6].

DTI performed at term equivalent age in 32 Extremely Low Birth Weight infants showed different FA values in white matter regions among infants with or without white matter abnormalities associated with prematurity and/or Cerebral Palsy (CP). Low FA values of Region of Interests in DTI are related with later development of spastic CP in preterm infants with white matter abnormalities [7].

In a study compared DTI in 10 full term neonates without brain injury and 22 neonates with hypoxic ischemic encephalopathy and concluded that DTI can quantify the white matter injury in neonates with hypoxic ischemic encephalopathy [8].

A systematic review of 19 studies showed that low FA values in white matter regions are associated with poorer scores on neurodevelopmental clinical assessments at follow up. This review showed DTI of the key white matter tracts not only identifies the extent of damage but also predict the neurodevelopmental outcome [9].

Another systematic review included 11 studies were DTI data of very preterm and moderate to late preterm neonates at their term equivalent age compared with term controls found that DTI showed statistically significant diffusion measures in the white matter of preterm neonates which is associated with neurodevelopmental disability in later life. Hence, DTI can be used as a prognostic tool for neurodevelopmental disability in preterm neonates [10].

6.3 Magnetic resonance angiography

Magnetic Resonance Angiography (MRA) is a specific type of MRI, in which the arteries are specifically looked without seeing the overlying tissues. MRA may or may not require contrast material depending on the vessels being scanned. MRA plays a key role in evaluation of neonatal arterial ischemic stroke (NAIS). MRA is able to find out the etiology of NAIS such as thrombus, embolism or cerebral vascular disorder like Moyamoya disease [11].

The below **Figure 4** showing narrowing of left middle cerebral artery in MRA.

6.4 Magnetic resonance venography

Magnetic Resonance Venography (MRV) is a type of MRI exam in which the veins are clearly visible without the overlying tissues and MRV often requires contrast material to enhance the visibility of veins. MRV is the gold standard investigation for diagnosing Cerebral Sinus Venous Thrombosis (CSVT). MRV used to diagnose CSVT in neonates underwent cardiac surgery and in neonates who received therapeutic hypothermia [12, 13].

6.5 Arterial spin labelling MRI

Arterial Spin Labelling (ASL) MRI is an advanced MRI technique used to assess the cerebral perfusion without the use of intravenous contrast. The protons of the intravascular arterial blood are labelled with radiofrequency pulses and that labelled protons are used as endogenous tracer to evaluate the brain perfusion [14].

Higher perfusion values in ASL MRI in neonates with HIE are associated with worse neurodevelopmental outcome. In a study done in 28 neonates with HIE, the median perfusion in basal ganglia and thalami was higher in neonates with adverse outcome than in

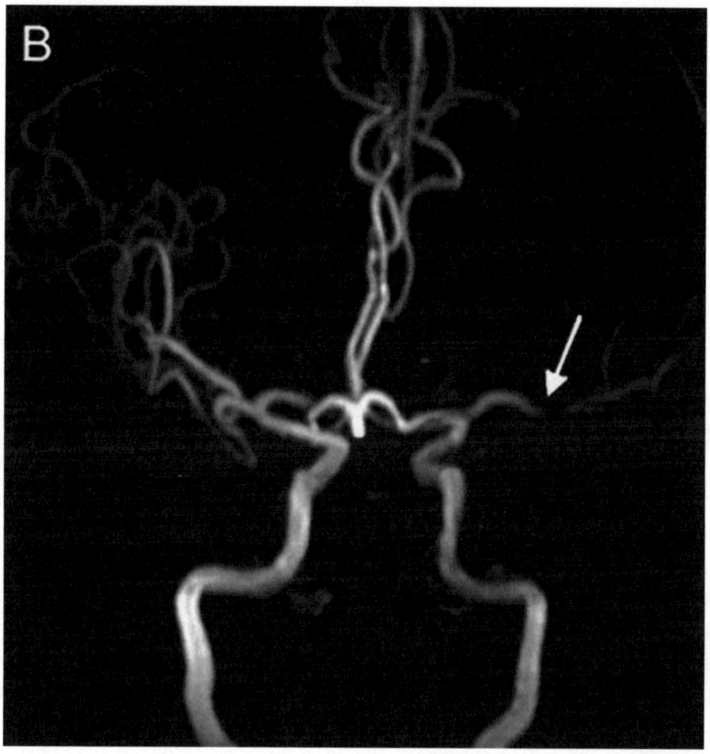

Figure 4.
Perinatal stroke MRA.

neonates with favourable outcome. ASL MRI can predict outcome in neonates with HIE. ASL MRI can add an extra element along with DWI and MRS in predicting the outcome in HIE. The combined information of ASL and MRS is the best predictor of outcome [15].

Brain growth and maturation is one of the most important processes that occur during the neonatal life. Advanced MRI tools such as DWI, DTI and ASL have been used to observe the process of brain maturation in neonates. ASL MRI provides quantitative measure of regional brain function and aging is associated with changes in regional brain function. ASL has been used to see changes in perfusion during the maturation of brain in neonates [16].

6.6 Phase contrast MRI

Phase-Contrast (PC) MRI is another technique of assessing the cerebral blood flow. PCMRI provides fast and reliable global cerebral blood flow measurement.

Even though ASL MRI can be used to assess cerebral blood flow, it is challenging particularly in neonates because it has low sensitivity, poor quantification and time consuming as it requires acquisition of several images repeatedly. Hence there is a need of alternative faster and more robust technique like phase contrast MRI arises [17].

The mean or global cerebral blood flow is assessed by dividing the total blood flow to the brain by brain volume. Phase Contrast Magnetic Resonance Angiography (PCMRA) used to measure blood flow in right and left internal carotid arteries and basilar artery, total blood flow to brain is calculated by sum of blood flow in right and left internal carotid arteries and basilar artery. Brain volume is determined by sum of volume of grey and white matter in cerebrum, cerebellum and brain stem.

In a study of 21 infants, the non-invasive PCMRI based method used to assess the mean cerebral blood flow (CBF). The mean cerebral blood flow is related to brain volume and postmenstrual age. The mean CBF increases postnatally in the first year of life [18].

Similar study was done in larger cohort of 344 infants, included 172 preterm infants and 172 term infants. This study concluded that mean CBF assessed by PCMRA is dependent on body weight and estimated brain weight also this mean CBF is more in term infants when compared to preterm infants at term equivalent age [19].

6.7 Magnetic resonance spectroscopy

Magnetic Resonance Spectroscopy (MRS) is more challenging than conventional MR imaging. Proton MRS works on the principle of detection of hydrogen nuclei in brain metabolites such as lactate, N-acetylaspartate (NAA), choline and creatine.

NAA a marker of neuronal activity. Choline, a marker for membrane turnover and myelination and Lactate, a marker of anaerobic respiration. NAA levels increase with brain maturity, but Choline and Lactate levels decrease with age as the rapid brain growth of the neonate slows down in infancy. Proton MRS used to assess these brain metabolite levels and thereby the brain maturation [20].

In a study done in 24 full term neonates with Hypoxic Ischemic Encephalopathy (HIE), conventional MR imaging and MRS was done, the differences of N-acetylaspartate / creatine (Cr), choline/Cr and lactate/Cr in the basal ganglia and thalamus in the HIE group were significantly different when compared to the control group, but there is no significant difference identified between mild to moderate HIE and severe HIE group. Hence MRS can be used as an additional tool for the diagnosis of HIE [21].

MRS used to assess the absolute concentration and concentration ratios of brain metabolites such as lactate (Lac), Creatine (Cr), N-acetylaspartate (NAA), and Choline (Cho), and to predict the outcome after hypoxic ischemic injury. Comparison of the mild HIE and severe HIE groups showed increased Lac/NAA and Lac/Cho and decreased NAA/Cr and NAA/Cho peak-area ratios, reduced NAA, and increased Lac in the infants with the worse outcome [22].

In a systematic review and meta-analysis of 32 studies of the prognostic accuracy of cerebral MRS biomarkers in infants with neonatal encephalopathy, concluded that deep gray matter Lac/NAA is the most accurate quantitative MRS biomarker within the neonatal period for prediction of neurodevelopmental outcome after NE [23].

MRS has been shown to detect abnormal accumulation of Lactate in brain parenchyma and CSF in patients with mitochondrial disorders. MRS provides a non-invasive tool for the diagnosis of mitochondrial diseases, especially in children with nonspecific findings on MRI, normal appearing MRI or a normal blood lactate/pyruvate ratio [24].

MRS shows elevated glycine levels in the brain of patients with Non Ketotic Hyperglycenemia [25]. Peroxisomal biogenesis disorder like Zellweger syndrome shows decreased NAA in proton MRS. Similarly in Pyruvate Dehydrogenase Complex deficiency MRS shows decreased NAA and Choline peak consistent with hypomyelination [26].

MRS has shown to be beneficial in diagnosing neuro metabolic disorders, mitochondrial disorders, diagnosis of HIE also in predicting the outcome after hypoxic ischemic injury and in assessing brain maturation.

7. Role of MRI in predicting neurodevelopmental outcome

MRI is used to predict neurodevelopmental outcome in term and preterm neonates.

7.1 MRI in prediction of neurodevelopmental outcome in term neonates with HIE

MRI is used to predict the outcome in term neonates after HIE. Several scoring systems developed over the past decades based on the injury pattern in MRI. A study done in 51 infants in whom MRI was done and their neurodevelopmental outcome was assessed at end of 3 months and 12 months. Score was assigned based on injury patterns in basal ganglia (BG), watershed (W), Basal ganglia / watershed (BG/W). Maximum score was assigned if the injury is more extensive. This study concluded that BG/W score was able to accurately predict good and poor neuromotor and cognitive outcome [27].

A study of 20 neonates with simplified MRI criteria was used to predict the outcome in term neonates with HIE. The MRI injury pattern was graded as follows,

- Grade 1—cases with no central and less than 10% peripheral change
- Grade 2—those with less than 30% central and/or 10–30% peripheral area change, and
- Grade 3—those with more than 30% central or peripheral change

This study showed that all neonates with grade 3 MRI changes were died or had poor neurodevelopmental outcome, grade 1 MRI changes had normal outcome and those with grade 2 MRI changes had moderate or normal outcome, and concluded that this simplified MRI criteria is highly predictive of neurodevelopmental outcome [28].

A study done by the National Institute of Child Health and Human Development (NICHD) Neonatal Research Network assessed the ability of MRI patterns of neonatal brain injury to predict death or Intelligent Quotient (IQ) at 6–7 years of age in infants who received hypothermia treatment for neonatal encephalopathy. The NICHD classified the injury pattern as follows:

- 0—normal MRI
- 1A—minimal cerebral lesions only with no involvement of Basal ganglia Thalami (BGT), Anterior Limb of Internal Capsule (ALIC), Posterior Limb of Internal Capsule (PLIC), or Watershed (WS) infarction
- 1B—more extensive cerebral lesions only with no involvement of BGT, ALIC, PLIC, or WS infarction
- 2A—any BGT, ALIC, PLIC, or WS infarction noted without any other cerebral lesions

- 2B—involvement of either BGT, ALIC, PLIC, or area of infarction and additional cerebral lesions and

- 3—Cerebral hemispheric devastation

The primary outcome was death or IQ <70. The disability among survivors also classified as mild, moderate and severe based on IQ score and Gross Motor Function classification system. This study concluded that 2B and 3 pattern of MRI injury is highly predictive of death or IQ <70 at 6–7years of age [29].

Similar scoring system based on MRI injury pattern also predicted the neurodevelopmental outcome at 18–24 months in neonates with HIE [30].

Even though grading systems vary, but the MRI injury patterns after neonatal hypoxic ischemic encephalopathy used to predict the future neurodevelopmental outcomes.

7.2 MRI in predicting the neurodevelopmental outcome in Preterm neonates

Preterm neonates who are born at gestational age of 32 weeks or less are more at risk of adverse neurodevelopmental outcomes. MRI at term equivalent age has been used to predict the neurodevelopmental outcome in preterm neonates.

A study done in 167 very preterm infants found that moderate to severe white matter abnormalities in MRI at term equivalent age is predictive of adverse outcomes like cognitive delay, motor delay, cerebral palsy and neurosensory impairment at 2 years of age [31].

A systematic review of 20 studies showed that the presence of moderate to severe white matter abnormalities on MRI around term equivalent age can predict the motor function and cerebral palsy in very preterm infants [32].

8. Conclusions

Neuroimaging is essential in evaluation of neonates with encephalopathy and other neurological problems. Even though CUS and CT scan also commonly used imaging modalities, MRI is more advantageous in terms of superior image quality and it provides multiple tissue parameters like location, extent, vascularity and functional status. MRI avoids the risk of exposure to ionizing radiation. MRI is the imaging of choice for better delineation of posterior fossa structures. Newer modalities of MRI like DWI, DTI, and MRS are used to accurately assess the anatomy and functional status of brain, also to predict the neurodevelopmental outcome.

The only disadvantage of MRI is requirement of stronger magnetic field and longer image acquisition time, which is a major hindrance in doing MRI in critically ill neonates. When we suspect intracranial hemorrhage in term neonates with encephalopathy, a non contrast CT scan can be done. But with the availability of safer MRI technique, with the advent of newer MRI techniques and also with the availability of MRI compatible instruments, MRI scan could be considered as initial imaging modality even in sick neonates for better assessment.

DOI: http://dx.doi.org/10.5772/intechopen.109479

Author details

Manikandasamy Veluchamy
Department of Neonatology, NMC Royal Women's Hospital, Abu Dhabi, United Arab Emirates

*Address all correspondence to: bharathi4samy@gmail.com

References

[1] Rumack CM, Johnson ML. Role of computed tomography and ultrasound in neonatal brain imaging. The Journal of Computed Tomography. 1983;**7**(1):17-29

[2] Chau V, Poskitt KJ, Sargent MA, Lupton BA, Hill A, Roland E, et al. Comparison of computer tomography and magnetic resonance imaging scans on the third day of life in term newborns with neonatal encephalopathy. Pediatrics. 2009;**123**(1):319-326

[3] Poretti A, Blaser SI, Lequin MH, Fatemi A, Meoded A, Northington FJ, et al. Neonatal neuroimaging findings in inborn errors of metabolism. Journal of Magnetic Resonance Imaging. 2013;**37**(2):294-312

[4] Mader I, Schöning M, Klose U, Küker W. Neonatal cerebral infarction diagnosed by diffusion-weighted MRI: Pseudonormalization occurs early. Stroke. 2002;**33**(4):1142-1145

[5] Vermeulen RJ et al. Diffusion-weighted and conventional MR imaging in neonatal hypoxic ischemia: Two-year follow-up study. Radiology. 2008;**249**(2):631-639

[6] Feng K, Rowell AC, Andres A, Bellando BJ, Lou X, Glasier CM, et al. Diffusion tensor MRI of white matter of healthy full-term newborns: Relationship to neurodevelopmental outcomes. Radiology. 2019;**292**(1):179-187

[7] Kim D-Y, Park H-K, Kim N-S, Hwang S-J, Lee HJ. Neonatal diffusion tensor brain imaging predicts later motor outcome in preterm neonates with white matter abnormalities. Italian Journal of Pediatrics. 2016;**42**(1):104

[8] Li H-X, Feng X, Wang Q, Dong X, Yu M, Tu W-J. Diffusion tensor imaging assesses white matter injury in neonates with hypoxic-ischemic encephalopathy. Neural Regeneration Research. 2017;**12**(4):603-609

[9] Dibble M, O'Dea MI, Hurley T, Byrne A, Colleran G, Molloy EJ, et al. Diffusion tensor imaging in neonatal encephalopathy: A systematic review. Archives of Disease in Childhood. Fetal and Neonatal Edition. 2020;**105**(5):480-488

[10] Dibble M, Ang JZ, Mariga L, Molloy EJ, Bokde ALW. Diffusion tensor imaging in very preterm, moderate-late preterm and term-born neonates: A systematic review. The Journal of Pediatrics. 2021;**232**:48-58.e3

[11] Husson B, Hertz-Pannier L, Adamsbaum C, Renaud C, Presles E, Dinomais M, et al. MR angiography findings in infants with neonatal arterial ischemic stroke in the middle cerebral artery territory: A prospective study using circle of Willis MR angiography. European Journal of Radiology. 2016;**85**(7):1329-1335

[12] Claessens NHP, Algra SO, Jansen NJG, Groenendaal F, de Wit E, Wilbrink AA, et al. Clinical and neuroimaging characteristics of cerebral sinovenous thrombosis in neonates undergoing cardiac surgery. The Journal of Thoracic and Cardiovascular Surgery. 2018;**155**(3):1150-1158

[13] Munster CB, El-Shibiny H, Szakmar E, Yang E, Walsh BH, Inder TE, et al. Magnetic resonance venography to evaluate cerebral sinovenous thrombosis in infants receiving therapeutic hypothermia. Pediatric Research. 19 Jul 2022. [Epub ahead of print] PMID: 35854084

[14] Petersen ET, Zimine I, Ho Y-CL, Golay X. Non-invasive measurement

of perfusion: A critical review of arterial spin labelling techniques. The British Journal of Radiology. 2006;**79**(944):688-701

[15] De Vis JB, Hendrikse J, Petersen ET, de Vries LS, van Bel F, Alderliesten T, et al. Arterial spin-labelling perfusion MRI and outcome in neonates with hypoxic-ischemic encephalopathy. European Radiology. 2015;**25**(1):113-121

[16] Kim HG, Lee JH, Choi JW, Han M, Gho S-M, Moon Y. Multidelay arterial spin-labeling MRI in neonates and infants: Cerebral perfusion changes during brain maturation. AJNR. American Journal of Neuroradiology. 2018;**39**(10):1912-1918

[17] Liu P, Qi Y, Lin Z, Guo Q, Wang X, Lu H. Assessment of cerebral blood flow in neonates and infants: A phase-contrast MRI study. NeuroImage. 2019;**185**:926-933

[18] Varela M, Groves AM, Arichi T, Hajnal JV. Mean cerebral blood flow measurements using phase contrast MRI in the first year of life: MEAN CBF IN FIRST YEAR OF LIFE. NMR in Biomedicine. 2012;**25**(9):1063-1072

[19] Wagenaar N, Rijsman LH, Nieuwets A, Groenendaal F, NeoQflow Study Group. Cerebral blood flow measured by phase-contrast magnetic resonance angiography in preterm and term neonates. Neonatology. 2019;**115**(3):226-233

[20] Xu D, Bonifacio SL, Charlton NN, et al. MR spectroscopy of normative premature newborns. Journal of Magnetic Resonance Imaging. 2011;**33**(2):306-311

[21] Guo L, Wang D, Bo G, Zhang H, Tao W, Shi Y. Early identification of hypoxic-ischemic encephalopathy by combination of magnetic resonance (MR) imaging and proton MR spectroscopy. Experimental and Therapeutic Medicine. 2016;**12**(5): 2835-2842

[22] Cheong JLY, Cady EB, Penrice J, Wyatt JS, Cox IJ, Robertson NJ. Proton MR spectroscopy in neonates with perinatal cerebral hypoxic-ischemic injury: Metabolite peak-area ratios, relaxation times, and absolute concentrations. AJNR. American Journal of Neuroradiology. 2006;**27**(7):1546-1554

[23] Thayyil S, Chandrasekaran M, Taylor A, Bainbridge A, Cady EB, Chong WKK, et al. Cerebral magnetic resonance biomarkers in neonatal encephalopathy: A meta-analysis. Pediatrics. 2010;**125**(2):e382-e395

[24] ElBeheiry AA, Abougabal AM, Omar TI, Etaby AN. Role of brain magnetic resonance spectroscopy in the evaluation of suspected mitochondrial diseases in children: Experience in 30 pediatric cases. Egyptian Journal of Radiology and Nuclear Medicine. 2014;**45**(2):523-533

[25] Nicolasjilwan M, Ozer H, Wintermark M, Matsumoto J. Neonatal non-ketotic hyperglycinemia. Journal of Neuroradiology. 2011;**38**(4):246-250

[26] Ah Mew N, Loewenstein JB, KadomN, Lichter-KoneckiU, GropmanAL, Martin JM, et al. MRI features of 4 female patients with pyruvate dehydrogenase E1 alpha deficiency. Pediatric Neurology. 19 Jul 2011;**45**(1):57-59. PMID:35854084 [Epub ahead of print]

[27] Barkovich AJ, Hajnal BL, Vigneron D, Sola A, Partridge JC, Allen F, et al. Prediction of neuromotor outcome in perinatal asphyxia: Evaluation of MR scoring systems. AJNR. American Journal of Neuroradiology. 1998;**19**(1):143-149

[28] Jyoti R, O'Neil R, Hurrion E. Predicting outcome in term neonates with hypoxic-ischaemic encephalopathy using simplified MR criteria. Pediatric Radiology. 2006;**36**(1):38-42

[29] Shankaran S, McDonald SA, Laptook AR, Hintz SR, Barnes PD, Das A, et al. Neonatal magnetic resonance imaging pattern of brain injury as a biomarker of childhood outcomes following a trial of hypothermia for neonatal hypoxic-ischemic encephalopathy. The Journal of Pediatrics. 2015;**167**(5):987-993.e3

[30] Trivedi SB, Vesoulis ZA, Rao R, Liao SM, Shimony JS, McKinstry RC, et al. A validated clinical MRI injury scoring system in neonatal hypoxic-ischemic encephalopathy. Pediatric Radiology. 2017;**47**(11):1491-1499

[31] Woodward LJ, Anderson PJ, Austin NC, Howard K, Inder TE. Neonatal MRI to predict neurodevelopmental outcomes in preterm infants. The New England Journal of Medicine. 2006;**355**(7):685-694

[32] van Hooft J, van der Lee JH, Opmeer BC, CSH A-M, AGE L, BWJ M, et al. Predicting developmental outcomes in premature infants by term equivalent MRI: Systematic review and meta-analysis. Systematic Reviews. 2015;**4**(1):71

Chapter 6

Advances in Magnetic Resonance Imaging in Multiple Sclerosis

Rasha Abdel-Fahim

Abstract

Multiple sclerosis is the second most common cause of disability in young adults. Conventional imaging so far failed to explain the extent of clinical disability even by careful examination of white matter lesion volume and their topographical distribution. The increasing availability of ultra-high field imaging allowed the improvement in understanding the dynamic lesional and extralesional pathology in different stages of the disease and their potential contribution to clinical and cognitive disability. The contribution of cortical lesions of different subtypes, the degree of microstructural damage in those lesions has been examined. This is in addition to the influence of white matter lesions and spinal cord pathology on the degree of disability in multiple sclerosis. Prognostic factors influencing long-term disability in patients with multiple sclerosis have also been a subject of interest for many years, particularly their significance in early decision-making with regard to disease-modifying treatment choice and early initiation. The frequency of iron rims in white matter lesions has been linked to increased disease severity in multiple sclerosis. Iron rim lesions' potential evolution to slowly expanding lesions as well as the long-term prognostic impact of such lesions on the degree of clinical disability has also been examined in this chapter.

Keywords: cortical lesions, multiple sclerosis, iron rims, slowly expanding lesions, magnetization transfer imaging

1. Introduction

Multiple sclerosis (MS) is a chronic inflammatory disease of the nervous system, and it is the second commonest cause of disability in young adults. It presents with different phenotypes, the commonest being relapsing remitting which presents with relapses, and it constitutes around 80% of patients. Most patients in the relapsing–remitting phase convert to the secondary progressive phase between 10 and 15 years from onset. During the secondary progressive phase of the disease, the clinical decline is usually gradual with some patients experiencing superimposed relapses. A cohort of patients, of around 15%, presents in a progressive phase from onset and labeled as primary progressive MS (PPMS).

Magnetic resonance imaging (MRI) is very significant not only in diagnosis but also in providing prognostic views. Utilization of MRI in diagnosis has depended mainly on white matter (WM) lesion load as well as spatial distribution and temporal accumulation to establish dissemination in space and time.

Despite advances in imaging, extensive examination of WM lesions over the years has not explained the variability in clinical course and the variable degree of physical and cognitive disability posing an obvious struggle to address the clinico-radiological paradox.

The evolution of MRI techniques over the years and more recent advances in high and ultra-high-field imaging has contributed significantly to bridging the gap between radiological, clinical, and even pathological views in MS. This has provided a paramount insight into lesions pathology and in turn MS pathology.

Recent evolution of imaging in MS has focused on exploring imaging techniques that could explain clinical disability given that WM lesions solely cannot account fully for the clinical decline. In turn, such understanding of mechanisms of MS pathology could facilitate prognostic tools which would be a useful biomarker in decision-making with regards to disease-modifying treatment (DMT) initiation.

2. Cortical gray matter pathology in MS

Cortical lesion pathology is an emerging imaging biomarker that has been receiving an increasing attention due to its increasingly perceived contribution to clinical disability.

Cortical lesions are prevalent at the early stages of MS disease course and their abundance has been illustrated in early MRI and histology studies on post-mortem MS brains [1]. It is suggested that they develop in the early stages of the disease even before (WM) lesions [2].

Despite their significant contribution to MS pathology and physical and cognitive disability, their consideration during decision-making is non-existent. This is due to the current challenge in detecting cortical lesions using clinical scanners and the need for higher magnetic field strength to facilitate their depiction.

3. Cortical lesions pathology in MS

Cortical lesions are classified based on their location within the cortex into type 1 (Leukocortical) which extend between the cortex and white matter, type 2 (intra-cortical) which are usually confined to the cortex, and type 3 (subpial) which usually extend from the pia surface to cortical layer 3 or 4 and usually appear as ribbon-like lesions extending through large surface of the cortex [3]. Leukocortical lesions are usually the most prevalent type of cortical lesions, accounting for over 60% of the total cortical lesions count (**Figures 1** and **2**) [4].

Pathology of either cortical lesions or WM lesions development is complex, has been hypothesized over the years, and is likely to involve multiple mechanisms. Spinal lesion load correlated to subpial lesion subtypes despite small WM lesion load, suggesting a similar mechanism of lesion development with their proximity to the meninges [6, 7]. A difference in the intensity of lesions in the cortex from WM lesions in 7Tesla T2* was noted, which could reflect pathology finding of less inflammation in cortical lesions in comparison with WM lesions and supports the notion that they have different mechanisms, degree of tissue damage, and probably contribute to disability in different ways [3, 6].

The small size of cortical lesions and the scarcity of myelin in the cortex posed challenges to their detection via conventional clinical magnetic resonance imaging tools. However, advancement in the magnetic imaging field, especially different

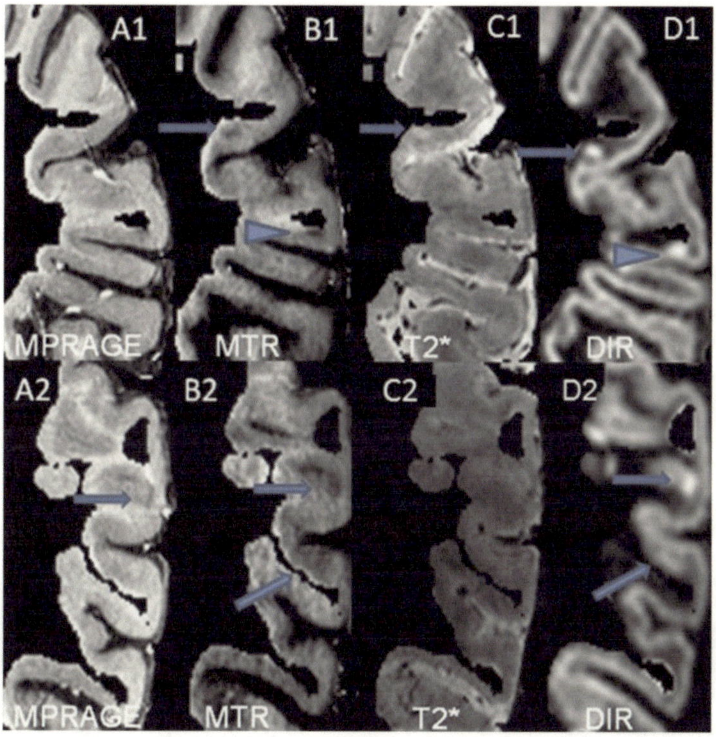

Figure 1.
Cortical lesions as seen in different sequences. To ensure blinding, the white matter was erased and lesion detection was undertaken using the segmented cortical ribbon. MTR offers advantages in providing increased sensitivity in GM lesion detection and more clear classification of lesion location. Intracortical lesions (arrows) and mixed leukocortical lesions (arrow heads) were detected on MTR (B1, B2) and DIR (D1, D2) but were undetectable on MPRAGE (A1, A2) or T2 (C1, C2). DIR (arrows D1) frequently misclassified lesions as leukocortical when MTR maps (arrows B1) clearly show intracortical lesion with normal appearing adjacent WM [5].*

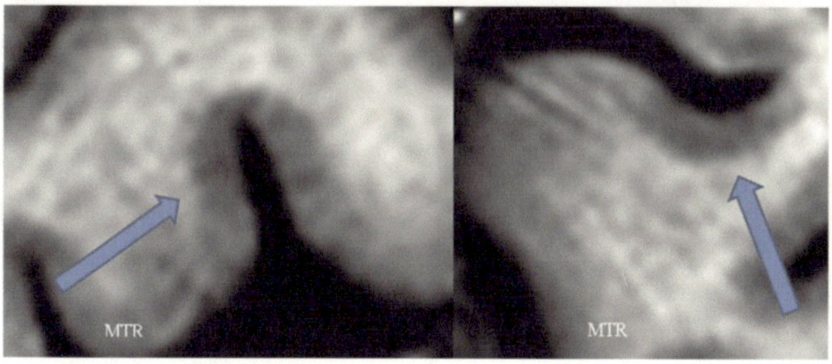

Figure 2.
Examples of subpial cortical lesions (arrows) on MTR [5].

sequences, as well as ultra-high field strength, facilitated further studying of cortical lesions and their contribution to understanding MS clinical course.

Ultra-high-field imaging at 7 Tesla has improved our understanding of cortical pathology via its increased sensitivity to depicting cortical lesions in comparison with 3 T MRI sequences. Magnetization transfer imaging (MTI), magnetization prepared two rapid acquisition gradient echo (MP2RAGE), T2*, and Double inversion recovery (DIR) sequences at 7 Tesla proved sensitive to depicting cortical lesions *in vivo*, particularly leukocortical lesions, however, with less sensitivity to intracortical and subpial lesions [5, 8–10]. DIR, phase-sensitive inversion recovery (PSIR), and MP2RAGE have proven less sensitive to cortical lesions depiction in comparison with 7 T PSIR, MP2RAGE, T2*, and MTR especially of subpial subtype (**Figure 3**) [5, 8, 11].

Cortical lesion load, especially leukocortical lesions, is generally higher in patients with SPMS in comparison with those in RRMS. However, no significant difference was observed in intracortical or subpial lesion load among different MS phenotypes [6]. Higher cortical lesion load was the main difference between progressive and relapsing cohort even on comparing WM and spinal cord lesion load, favoring the correlation between focal cortical lesion pathology and progressive phase of the disease [6]. Cortical lesion load was higher in those with higher WM lesion loads; leukocortical lesion load in particular correlated with WM lesions load with less correlation indicated with other cortical lesions subtypes [6].

To determine factors influencing the degree of disability in MS patients, the main emphasis should not only be on cortical lesion load but also the topographical

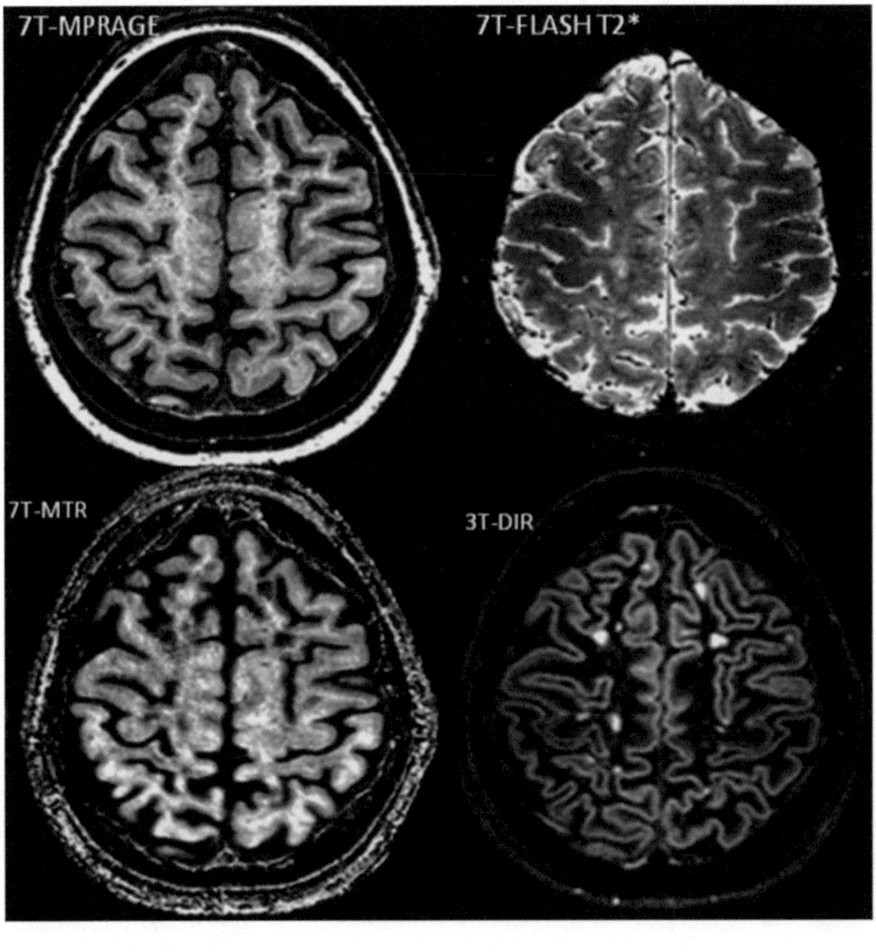

Figure 3.
Axial view of the sequences used in a relapsing–remitting MS patient [5].

distribution of those lesions. Utilizing ultra-high field strength allowed not only improved sensitivity in detecting cortical lesions but also better characterization of their topographical distribution. Cortical lesions tend to have a predilection to motor areas such as premotor cortex, precentral gyrus, and mesial temporal regions [10, 12]. However, it is important to appreciate technical challenges when using ultra-high field imaging to assess cortical lesions as it often underestimates lesion load in temporal and occipital lobes due to associated inhomogeneity observed in those areas at higher magnetic field strength.

4. Cortical lesions and clinical disability in MS

The impact of cortical lesions on physical and cognitive disability has been a subject of interest and extensively examined. Studies revealed a higher number of cortical lesions in patients with progressive MS in comparison with those with relapsing–remitting MS (RRMS), as well as association between worsening physical disability indicated by EDSS and cortical lesion load especially subpial lesions [13]. On the other hand, cognitive performance showed a higher association with leukocortical lesion load, subpial lesion load, and cortical thickness, but the association with leukocortical lesion and subpial lesion load was stronger than with cortical thickness at 7 Tesla imaging [13]. Another study observed that cortical lesions T1 values were not different in RRMS patients in comparison with progressive MS patients, but they were higher in leukocortical lesions in comparison with other cortical lesions subtypes [6].

Using DIR at 1.5 T, analysis of cortical lesion load at baseline correlated with the degree of physical disability, indicated by EDSS, 5 years later, with no significant contribution to the rate of new lesions development. Furthermore, there was no difference in the rate of development of cortical lesions in different disease phenotypes. This could well be due to the lower sensitivity of DIR at 1.5 T to cortical lesions detection [14]. Taking into consideration WM lesion load as well as degree of gray matter atrophy, the association of cortical lesions with cognitive and physical disability in all MS disease phenotypes was more consistent than any other parameters [14].

Improved and early detection of cortical lesions would contribute significantly to earlier consideration of diagnosis, potentially providing a step closer to being considered in diagnostic criteria, and potential implications on prognosis especially on physical and cognitive outcomes. Most importantly, improved imaging detection of cortical lesions would offer a promising biomarker for DMTs evolution and treatment targets.

5. Role of automated lesion detection

Manual segmentation of lesions is time-consuming and subject to inter as well as intra-rater variability. Automated detection of cortical lesions on MRI has been evolving in recent years. However, implementation of deep learning methods in cortical lesions segmentation has been challenging due to the difficulty in detecting some lesion subtypes, especially subpial and intracortical lesions, in addition to the relatively small size of cortical lesions and the lower contrast in comparison with surrounding normal-appearing gray matter tissue. High magnetic field strengths such as 3 T and 7 T are often needed to facilitate cortical lesion detection. Despite higher field strength providing better resolution and signal-to-noise ratio, it has higher field inhomogeneity across the images in comparison with conventional imaging, which poses a challenge to implementing automated segmentation techniques.

Multiple sclerosis lesion analysis at seven tesla (MSLAST) is a new automated method to detect lesions based on estimation of partial volume and topographical constraints using a single MP2RAGE, which provides good tissue contrast for detection of WM as well as cortical lesions and less affected by B0 and B1 inhomogeneities. Automated segmentation using a single image MP2RAGE showed better performance with WM lesion detection than cortical lesions detection, with sensitivity at 74% and 58%, respectively, and false positive rate at 40%. When the radiological MS lesions definition (volume approximately ≥15 ul) was implemented, its detection rate improved to 80% of WM lesions and 63% of cortical lesions [15].

Automated segmentation was reproducible than manual segmentation, however, with significant challenges, in particular using MSLAST technique, such as the lack of sensitivity to detect periventricular lesions as they have similar contrast to CSF, hence were included in the CSF mask. The same hurdle is noted with cortical lesion segmentation due to the lack of strong contrast between gray matter and cortical lesions, as well as the small size of cortical lesions. MSLAST also underestimated lesions volume, probably due to the partial volume effect and its lack of efficiency in delineating lesions borders [15].

Working on the range of sequences available at 7 T and improving the tissue contrast will help achieve better brain segmentation, partial volume estimation, and lesion segmentation, which in turn will improve the quality of MSLAST technique and its accuracy.

The second method of automated lesion detection at 7 Tesla using MP2RAGE and T2* sequences showed cortical lesion detection rate was 67%, false positive rate was relatively high at 42%, however, with retrospect analysis by a second reviewer false positives were deemed to be potential lesions [16]. This supports the notion of how challenging cortical lesion segmentation could prove.

A relatively new deep learning-based method is Cortical Lesions AI-based Assessment in Multiple Sclerosis (CLAIMS) which compared cortical lesion detection rates using ultra-high field 7 T MP2RAGE and T2*w contrasts (T2* EPI and T2* GRE) fed into their U-net based deep learning method. It showed that T2*w sequences did not add any value to the sensitivity of cortical lesion detection. Furthermore, they showed that models utilized T2*w sequences either T2* EPI or T2* GRE performed very poorly in comparison with models that used only MP2RAGE. Intracortical lesion subtype detection, as expected, was the most challenging with a detection rate of 53%, while performance was better for subpial and leukocortical lesions with a detection rate of 70% and 80%, respectively. CLAIMS also compared models with MP2RAGE of different voxel size at 0.5 mm or 0.7 mm or both 0.5 mm and 0.7 mm. They found that lesion detection rate dropped by 20% on moving from 0.5 mm acquisitions to 0.7 mm acquisitions which confers the importance of higher resolution images for lesion detection rate, even using automated methods of image analysis [17].

On comparing CLAIMS and MSLAST, CLAIMS showed higher performance with a good degree of classification of cortical lesions to intracortical and leukocortical [17].

Despite intense efforts and increasingly sophisticated techniques in automated lesion detection methods, intracortical lesion detection remains poor, as well as overall false positive rates. The lesser contrast between cortical lesions and their surrounding normal-appearing tissue in comparison with WM lesions and their surrounding tissue constitutes a challenge to a highly accurate deep-based learning method to be utilized reliably in cortical lesion detection.

6. Progression independent of relapses (PIRA)

Progression independent of relapses (PIRA) is an increasingly recognized phenomenon in MS, particularly in the progressive phase of the disease but also in RRMS patients [18]. Studies on the correlation between MS relapses and associated new T2 lesions with disability progression are controversial. Some suggest that the frequency of relapses in early disease course influences long-term disability progression [19], while recent studies did not identify such a correlation [18].

Ocrelizumab appeared to be superior to Betaferon in reducing PIRA as well as reducing the frequency of relapses, explaining why Ocrelizumab is effective in primary progressive MS patients [20]. In the same study, PIRA was observed to account for 80–90% of disability progression [20].

The frequency of new lesions was found to be higher in patients who had progression related to relapses (90%) than in those with PIRA (11%), however, lesion accrual in the PIRA group was identified a few years before disability progression refuting the theory that progression is due to new lesion accrual [21]. Despite the evolution in DMTs, reducing the risk of relapses associated with disability, it did not significantly influence the risk of PIRA which increased with the age of onset of disease and with spinal cord lesions [21].

7. No evidence of disease activity (NEDA)

The use of relapse rate as an outcome measure in MS trials is becoming increasingly irrelevant as it provides a very limited insight into the natural history of the disease and in turn DMTs efficacy.

The use of composite outcome measures that incorporate imaging with clinical data has proven to be more promising in monitoring disease evolution and treatment response in clinical trials. NEDA is a concept that developed over time, states no evidence of disease activity in terms of relapse, disability progression (defined as an increase in EDSS score of 1.5 points from a baseline score of 0, of 1.0 points from a baseline score of 1.0 to 5, or of 0.5 points from a baseline score of greater than 5.0), or MRI activity (NEDA-3) is an increasingly used composite outcome measure to assess disease evolution in clinical trials. With further incorporation of imaging into this composite, NEDA-4 was introduced. NEDA-4 adds whole brain volume loss (mean annualized rate of brain volume loss in healthy brains should be less than 0.4%) to NEDA-3 measures [22].

Even though achieving NEDA-3 in the first 2 years of disease onset was not found to influence long-term progression [21], achieving NEDA-4 was correlated with reduced risk of long-term progression [23] which is compatible with the long-acknowledged view of the role of brain atrophy in long-term disease progression [18].

Despite the advantages around using a composite scale incorporating different measures, there is some skepticism regards some of these scales especially EDSS. The non-linear progression of this scale, the non-uniform progression between different stages, and the inter and intra-assessor variability when implementing at different clinical visits. It is also not easy to implement and imprecise at the lower end of the scale, too driven by mobility distances at the middle and higher end of the scale and fails to take into account upper limb function which means a patient can score very highly for having one severe cord relapse ending the patient wheelchair dependent [24–26].

It is also important to note that despite the NEDA being a vital tool in monitoring disease outcomes, it mainly evaluates the active aspect of the disease without much emphasis on the neurodegenerative aspect [27]. Given that cognitive decline constitutes a significant aspect of MS disease, and it usually represents one of the earliest signs of disease progression and the degenerative component of MS, it will be crucial that it is taken into account in such composite scales [27].

8. Iron rim and slowly expanding lesions

Prognostic scores have been an area of interest for decades. Prognostic factors employ a mix of clinical features or MRI metrics. However, current radiological prognostic metrics depend on the presence of a higher degree of tissue damage to predict long-term severe disability. Hence targeting those patients with high-efficacy treatments at that stage of the disease, when a lot of the damage is already established, is probably not the most effective way of preventing future disability. It is also important to note that application of various prognostic indicators is challenging at the individual level and more acceptable at the group level.

With the continuous advancement in MS imaging field and the increase availability of ultra-high field imaging, it is important to be able to risk stratify MS patients early in the disease course, to assist DMT choice. In order to do this, we need an early radiological prognostic indicator to salvage brain tissue from future damage and improve brain reserve, which will be crucial when patients are entering the progressive stage of the disease.

Iron is the most abundant trace metal in healthy individuals' brains. Dysregulation of brain iron levels correlates to development of various neurodegenerative diseases, including the worsening of MS [28]. Iron is present in macrophages; however, its concentration varies depending on the stage of the disease. Histopathology showed that iron is present at high levels in slowly expanding lesions, but most importantly not present in remyelinating plaques [28].

Despite the controversies around brain iron accumulation and if it is contributing to neurodegeneration or if it is simply an epiphenomenon reflecting brain tissue degeneration, it is clear the association between its presence and worsening clinical parameters. It is even becoming more apparent as a prognostic factor.

Magnetic resonance imaging is sensitive to iron detection. T2 and T2* relaxation contrasts are shown to be sensitive to iron detection in comparison with T1 relaxation. In particular, T2* and susceptibility-weighted imaging (SWI) are more sensitive to iron detection than T2w. Iron enhancement increases with higher magnetic field strength. Despite how sensitive those parameters are to iron deposition, they do not reflect iron concentration, so they constitute a qualitative measure of iron presence. Magnetic field correlation imaging (MFC), phase imaging, and R2* mapping are semi-quantitative techniques that offer some rough quantification to iron content, but their estimates depend on iron content in a given voxel as well as iron content in voxels surrounding. Quantitative susceptibility mapping (QSM) uses GRE phase images and eliminates blooming artifacts to quantify the local tissue magnetic properties (**Figure 4**).

Iron rim WM lesions are reported to constitute between 10 and 15% of all WM lesions [29, 30]. Iron rims around WM lesions appearing as rim of elevated R2* using 7 T was found in a small cohort of patients of different disease phenotypes either RRMS or progressive MS and in patients with different degree of disability, which reflects the degree of heterogeneity in iron distribution in MS patients. Other studies showed that the core of white matter lesions had low R2* relaxation reflecting low myelin and iron, while R2* was high around the demyelinated core reflecting high myelin and iron deposition [31]. This pattern of iron deposition is also present in slowly expanding lesions [32].

A study using QSM at 7 T followed patients for 2.4 years showed no significant change in size or signal intensity pattern of WM lesions [33]. However, there was a change in characteristics of some of those lesions, mainly in terms of iron contents and distribution within those lesions [33]. This change in characteristics was explained by the interaction of different macrophages phenotypes, classically iron-rich activated macrophages with M1-polarization which secretes proin-flammatory toxic cytokines and are known to be neurotoxic, and M2-polarized macrophages which have the phagocytic capacity and are significant for tissue repair [34]. The change in iron distribution in some iron lesions or the switch from non-iron to iron at times is hypothesized to be due to the alteration in macrophages phenotypes [33].

On the other hand, iron rims in cortical lesions were investigated using 7 T T2* GRE and inversion recovery turbo field echo (TFE) sequences in post-mortem brains

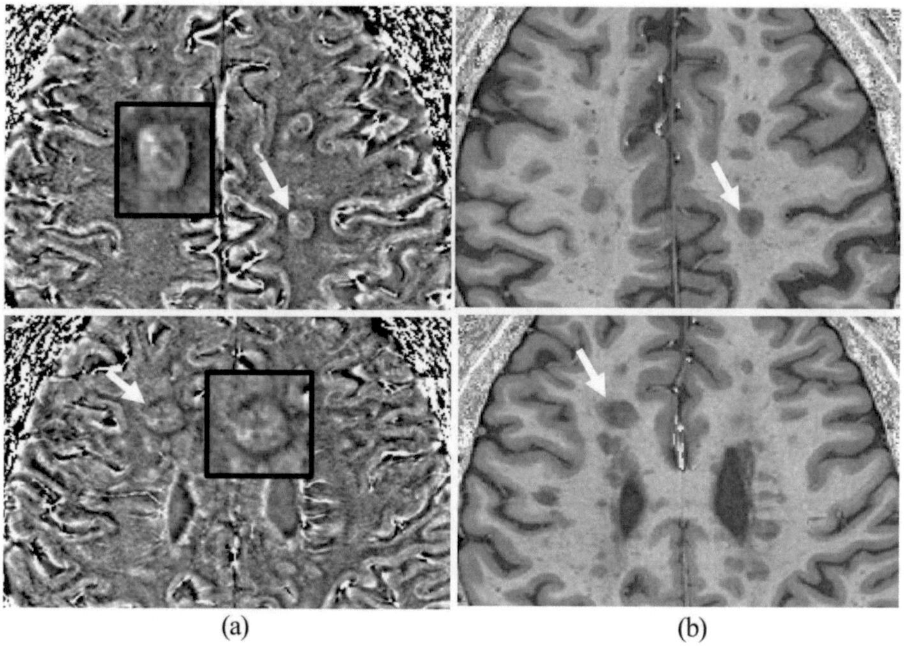

Figure 4.
Typical appearance of two lesions with rims on (a) SWI-filtered phase image corresponding with (b) T1-weighted (MPRAGE). Enlarged images of the lesions indicated using the white arrows from different patients are shown in the black box with the characteristic hypo-intense rim surrounding most of the lesion [5].

of MS patients. They found that iron rims lesions (IRLs) are associated with activated microglia at the border of chronic active cortical lesions and show high iron contents [10]. Another post-mortem imaging study that employed T2* maps at 7 T showed large areas of demyelination detected in histopathology, extending from the subpial surface across all layers of the cortex and involving full gyri in some sections, but often went undetected in imaging. Re-examining the images yielded 67% of the undetected lesions detected retrospectively. This disparity between imaging and histopathology was not solely due to the small size of lesions being difficult to detect, but also due to the variability of cortical ribbons contrast according to their function, which affects the contrast between lesions and surrounding normal cortical tissue [35]. However, in that study, no iron-positive lesion edges were detected in cortical lesions, but the study sample was very small to draw any decisive conclusions [35]. A larger post-mortem study observed that cortical lesions with rims of activated microglia were more prevalent in patients with early active disease, died at a younger age and were associated with a higher frequency of chronic active WM lesions [36].

9. Slowly expanding lesions (SELs)

White matter chronic active lesions are prevalent in MS patients and pathologically they are surrounded by iron-laden activated microglia/macrophages that expand in size over time due to continuous demyelination and axonal loss [37]. While MS is composed of relapses and disease progression, it is suggested that active lesions, which are more prevalent in early disease course, contribute to relapses, whereas smoldering slowly expanding lesions (SELs), which are more prevalent in progressive MS, are more associated with disease progression [37]. The frequency of smoldering plaques increased with a longer disease duration [37]. Chronic active lesions have a paramagnetic iron rim, and it showed an increase in size gradually over time with serial T1 and T2w images over years [38]. However, other short-term longitudinal studies over 2.5 years using 7 T T2* did not show expansion of iron rim lesions over time [39].

Another attempt to understand and assess the evolution of WM lesions with and without iron rim is by categorizing lesions into two groups according to the way they take up contrast; centrifugally enhancing lesions (inside-out dynamic contrast leakage) and centripetally enhancing lesions (outside in dynamic contrast leakage) [40]. At follow-up, 18 months later, none of the centrifugally enhancing lesions had a phase rim [40]. The larger the size of lesions at baseline the higher chance phase rims will persist at follow-up regardless of the contrast pattern at baseline [40]. Rim persistence was also associated with the least recovery of T1 intensity in those lesions over time, suggesting that it is likely that phase rim does not only reflect associated inflammation but also a degree of tissue damage [40].

The brain's response to the acute inflammatory process in active lesions is to contain it via immune-mediated process or astroglial reaction, and failure of these processes can break down blood–brain barrier manifesting as centripetal enhancing lesions, and infiltration of macrophages and activated microglia, reflected in early phase rim [40].

Monitoring the change in the size of lesions over time using the Jacobian determinant of the deformation between reference and follow-up scans, showed that patients with PPMS had a higher number of SELs in comparison with RRMS patients [41].

SELs had lower T1 intensity at baseline and a greater drop in T1 intensity over time in comparison with T2 lesions that did not show an increase in size [41].

10. Examining the destructive nature of iron rim lesions and SELs

Rim lesions are noted to be larger in size than non-rim lesions [29] which could be due to the destructive microstructural nature of those lesions with larger centre and more extensive area of axonal loss, or due to the expanding nature of those lesions which could account for their larger size and more destructive nature. Some studies suggest that lesions which are larger at baseline are more likely to expand at follow-up [40] and adopt a slowly expanding lesion pattern. However, we also need to consider that it could be that those rim lesions are simply less likely to shrink in comparison with non-rim lesions [29].

In a post-mortem study using 7 T sequences, it was observed that neither shadow plaques (fully remyelinated lesions) nor active lesions showed edge-related iron accumulation in microglia or macrophages [29]. Most MS lesions had a very low concentration of iron in the centre of lesions in comparison with surrounding white matter [29]. In that study, iron rim lesions were more likely to expand, whereas non-rim lesions were more likely to shrink [29]. Most shadow plaques did not show iron in their lesion edges [29, 40]. The lack of iron at the edges of active lesions was explained by the likelihood that myelin at the edge of active lesions is mainly taken by macrophages, which are mobile and eventually accumulate in perivascular spaces, while in SELs tissue debris are taken by microglia which are far less mobile and remain at lesion edges for prolonged periods of time constituting iron rims [29].

In histopathology studies, remyelinated lesions were often more vulnerable to recurrent demyelination than normal-appearing white matter. Recurrent slowly expanding demyelination, in previously demyelination affecting remyelinated areas, correlated with incomplete remyelination in progressive MS patients [42].

MP2RAGE is composed of a modified MPRAGE sequence to create two different images at different inversion times aiming to alleviate the inhomogeneity at a high magnetic field, which affects spatial resolution [43]. While T1 prolongation manifesting in black holes is accepted as a marker of severe axonal loss, changes in T1 relaxation are suggested to be a good quantitative marker of the degree of demyelination and remyelination *in vivo*, as myelin strongly determines T1 relaxation time in MS lesions [43, 44]. On acquiring quantitative T1 maps with MP2RAGE sequence at 7 T, long T1 relaxation lesions appeared as black holes on T1 images, while short T1 relaxation lesions appeared as iso-intense or hypo-intense to cortex, and lesions with long T1 relaxation and short T1 relaxation areas were categorized as mixed lesions [44]. Correlating imaging to histopathology, T1 time was longer in demyelinated than remyelinated lesions and correlated with severe axonal loss. 7 T MP2RAGE was a good marker to differentiate demyelinated from remyelinated lesions as well as mild from severe axonal loss with a good degree of sensitivity and specificity [44]. Visual inspection of 7 T MP2RAGE T1 maps was a good measure to qualitatively classify fully demyelinated, partially demyelinated, or remyelinated lesions [44]. In the same study, 48% of PRL were long T1 and a similar percentage of mixed T1 while only 4% short T1 relaxation; moreover, PRL status explained 78% of the variance in T1 relaxation time [29, 44].

In keeping with previous studies suggesting that remyelination capacity can be variable depending on the topographical distribution of lesions, long T1 relaxation lesions were mostly noted in the periventricular and juxtacortical white matter with subcortical lesions showing more capacity to evolve into short T1 relaxation, while juxtacortical and periventricular lesions more likely to evolve into long T1 relaxation [44, 45]. In terms of remyelination capacity, small lesions with shorter T1 time showed more repair than large lesions with similarly short T1 relaxation time [44, 46]. As expected, with higher age at the time of lesion formation, there was an associated increase in mean T1 lesion relaxation at 7 T follow-up, even on taking into account disease duration and disease-modifying treatment [44].

Supporting the view of the destructive nature of SEL, a 9-year follow-up study showed EDSS score worsening over the follow-up period in patients with ≥4 SELs and lower baseline MTR in SELs [47]. Another study showed worse EDSS and ARMSS (age-related multiple sclerosis severity) at 10 years follow-up in patients with ≥4 IRL (**Figure 5**) [48]. Conversion to SPMS and higher EDSS at 9 years follow-up was associated with lower baseline MTR of SELs and higher T1 signal intensity decline in SELs at 2 years follow-up when compared with baseline, reflecting the contribution of the degree of microstructural tissue damage to the degree of future disability [47]. As the aforementioned factors can overlap in influencing EDSS worsening, and similarly conversion to SPMS is usually associated with higher and worsening EDSS, multivariate analysis that took into account the contribution of baseline SELs MTR, the proportion of SELs among white matter lesions to EDSS worsening at 9 years follow-up, and SPMS conversion found that while both factors contributed to EDSS worsening, the model only retained baseline SELs MTR as an independent predictor to SPMS conversion [47].

Evaluation of the effect of disease DMT on the evolution of SELs is crucial yet limited. It was observed that patients on Fingolimod and Natalizumab had higher volume and number of SELs over 24 months period, however, rate was lower in Natalizumab patients suggesting higher efficacy [49]. Moreover, SELs showed lower MTR values and T1 intensity in comparison with non-SEL, while non-SELs exhibited more improvement in MTR values than SELs [49]. This supports the view of the destructive nature of SELs and the notion that the lesser the degree of damage in lesions the higher the chance of recovering with disease-modifying treatment.

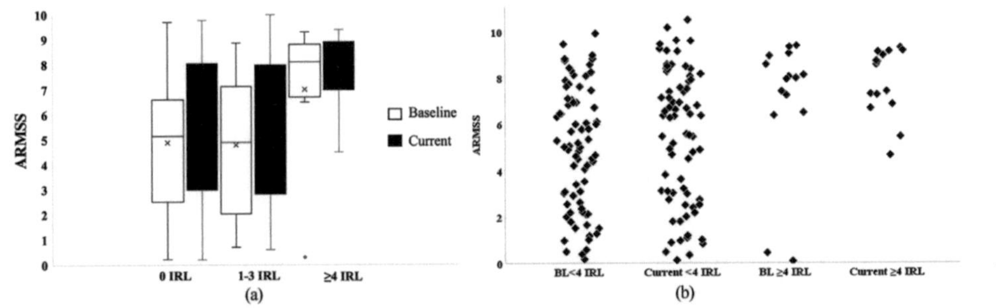

Figure 5.
ARMSS at baseline and current clinical follow-up in IRL patients. The number of IRLs were grouped to (a; 0 IRLs, 1–3 IRLs and ≥ 4 IRLs), (b; less than 4 IRLs and 4 or more rims) [5].

11. SELs and disability

Black holes have been a marker of neurodegeneration and axonal loss. The higher percentage of persistent black holes coincided with SELs; such an association suggests an evolution from an initial stage of chronic active lesions, or SELs to more chronic lesions, or black holes where severe axonal loss is the more prominent feature [50].

Chronic active lesions provide a reasonable explanation for clinical disability worsening in MS patients beyond mere total lesion load [50]. In a retrospective observational study with up to 12 years follow-up, employing a mixed-effects regression model observed that the increase in SELs predicted EDSS worsening not baseline total lesion volume or disease duration which were also included covariates in the model [50]. Moreover, for every unit increase in SELs, a fivefold higher risk for worsening EDSS; when paired with total baseline lesion volume in the same regression, the increase in SELs volume still performed better [50]. SELs log volumes negatively correlated with normalized brain volume and with normalized cortical gray matter [50].

It is thought that the neurodegenerative process in SELs is the main driver of physical disability in MS patients of different phenotypes. In PPMS patients on Ocrelizumab, the increase in T1 lesion volume between baseline and follow-up was less than that in PPMS patients not administering the drug [51]. Moreover, those on treatment had 5.1% of pre-existing T2 lesion volume identified as SELs, while those not on treatment had 7.1% [51]. Despite SELs accounting only for a small portion of T2 lesions, they accounted for a high proportion of T1 lesions developing in both groups of patients [51]. This indicates that the increase in T1 lesion burden in PPMS patients is due to chronic active disease activity and axonal tissue damage and it is predictive of clinical disease progression [51]. There was also a greater reduction in normalized T1 signal intensity in SELs regions in comparison with non-SEL regions in both groups [51]. Interestingly, neither whole brain volume loss nor new WM lesion formation predicted clinical disability progression in PPMS patients [51]. This suggests that chronic active lesions accumulation has a more predictive role in disability progression in PPMS patients than brain atrophy [51].

SPMS patients had greater, yet not significant, numbers of SELs in comparison with RRMS patients and had twofold greater T2 volume of SELs [52]. MTR values of SELs at baseline were lower than non-SELs in RRMS and SPMS patients and showed more decrease in their MTR values in comparison with non-SELs by the end of 72 weeks of study follow-up [52]. This suggests the severe tissue damage in SELs in comparison with non-SELs at baseline and their poor prognostic value earlier in the disease course, which would be of a significant value to guide treatment decisions early on in disease course.

MS lesions show a dynamic change in their microstructure mainly in the degree of active inflammation, demyelination, remyelination, or axonal loss. MS lesions detected on T2 sequences can evolve over time either increase in size or shrink. Various factors have been examined over the years to elucidate what contributes to the change in lesions size. This is significant as expanding lesions are thought to have an active edge contributing to their increase in size. Studying this further is relevant and significant as current DMTs in MS are mainly directed at targeting the active element of the disease, not disease progression. And as slowly expanding lesions are more prevalent in progressive MS and are thought to contribute to the progressive course of the disease, understanding its pathology further is crucial to evolve treatments for the progressive stage of the disease.

Taking available literature into consideration, we may need to look at DMTs from a different angle. All available treatments aim at new lesions development which is important for preventing relapses, however, gradual progression prevention seems far from achievable. In order to pave the way for progression prevention, further understanding of SELs as well as inactive lesions pathology is crucial as they are unlikely to remyelinate, and they correlate with worsening disability.

12. Brain volume

The average rate of yearly brain atrophy in a healthy individual is 0.1–0.4%, while it was estimated at 0.5–1.3% in MS patients [53]. There is a technical challenge in assessing brain volume in individual patients longitudinally, this is in addition to the presence of confounding factors such as the resolution of acute inflammation giving a false impression of volumetric brain atrophy, hence usually conclusions are more reliable when drawn on groups of patients rather than individuals. With higher magnetic field strength, it is less challenging examining volumetric brain measures in MS patients.

The correlation between cortical lesion load and cortical volume/thickness is controversial with some studies using DIR illustrating reduction in cortical thickness in patients who had cortical lesions in comparison with those with no visible cortical lesions [54], however, other studies using 7 T did not detect such a correlation either in individual cortical regions or in the cortex as a whole [6, 12].

Several studies showed the correlation of not only WM but also cortical gray matter atrophy with a physical disability at the early stages of the disease [55]. There is a consistent association found between the progressive stage of the disease and the reduction in cortical thickness, as well as a similar association observed between worsening disability and reduction in cortical thickness using 3 Tesla [13].

Gray matter fraction using DIR at 1.5 T showed lower gray matter volume at baseline in patients with progressive MS in comparison with those with relapsing–remitting MS, and the degree of volume loss over 5 years was higher in progressive patients in comparison with RRMS and benign MS patients. Furthermore, patients with higher cortical lesion load at baseline showed lower gray matter fraction in comparison with those with smaller cortical lesion load, and those who cumulated more cortical lesions had associated higher progression of their gray matter atrophy over the same number of years [14].

13. Spinal cord imaging

In pathology and radiology, the emphasis has mostly been on the cerebral involvement in MS with limited analysis of spinal cord involvement. The cervical spine has a predilection for involvement in MS. Spinal cord atrophy is more prevalent in progressive than relapsing MS patients and is considered as a reliable marker of progression in MS patients. Cord atrophy is more prominent in cervical than thoracic cord and shows a higher correlation to clinical disability parameters which supports the view that disease progression starts early in the disease course in RRMS patients and is not limited to the secondary progressive stage of the disease [56]. There was no correlation between the spinal cord lesion load and cord atrophy in all disease phenotypes which suggests that both factors contribute independently to the degree of disability [57].

PPMS patients usually have rapidly cumulating disability in comparison with RRMS patients and were not explained with lesion load which is usually higher in RRMS patients. Post-mortem studies showed an extensive axonal loss in spinal cord MS patients which reflects irreversible damage. Radiologically, cervical cord atrophy is a prominent consistent finding in patients with PPMS in comparison with RRMS patients and was even suggested as a tool to differentiate both phenotypes [58].

Due to technical challenges of cord imaging, image resolution, population variability, registration, and segmentation errors at the edge of the cord resulting in partial volume effect, it has been difficult to implement atrophy measures in clinical trials or indeed in clinical practice. Spinal cord atrophy assessments are mainly done via T1-weighted and T2*-weighted gradient-echo sequences, while methods for segmentation and atrophy calculation can be categorized into image based, intensity based, and surface based. Generalized boundary shift integral (GBSI) is a promising registration-based technique, which is based on BSI (boundary shift integral) but overcomes partial volume effects via measuring the percentage change in cord volume values directly from small intensity changes between images at the cord boundaries accounting for partial volume effects in these regions. As it quantifies spinal cord atrophy using direct estimates via registration-based measurement of cord atrophy, it improves sensitivity to variation in longitudinal volume changes. However, GBSI is very dependent on voxel size as it requires isotropic small voxels, and it also requires consistency between different time points to allow precision [59].

Various studies found the influence of spinal cord lesions on the degree of clinical disability extends beyond lesion load to topographical distribution. Furthermore, spinal cord lesions involving the central areas and the lateral funiculi of cervical spine were associated with a higher degree of disability indicated by EDSS [60]. Via implementing automated methods of assessing lesion distribution in different MS phenotypes and its correlation to disability suggested that RRMS patients show high lesion probability in the posterior column, while PPMS patients in the lateral and central cord and SPMS patients more in the posterior and lateral cord [60].

Limited spinal cord data are partially related to the challenging nature of spinal cord imaging with regards to the small mobile field of view contributing to increased likelihood of artefacts. The evolution of ultra-high-field imaging with the increase in signal-to-noise ratio and improved spatial resolution facilitated further examination of cervical cord pathology and potentially closer analysis of its potential pathogenesis. With histopathological studies suggesting outside-in pathological gradient mechanism of demyelination, describing the penetrating lymphocytes inducing inflammation via activating microglia and macrophages inducing focal demyelination [61]. In support of this theory, the use of 7 Tesla MRI imaging helped the accurate delineation of lesions in such a narrow eloquent space. It showed that spinal cord lesions are more frequent around the central canal as well as the CSF subpial interface, with higher frequency around the outer subpial portion of the cord early in the disease course in RRMS patients and move towards the centre around the central canal in SPMS patients [62]. This reflects the difference in dynamics of MS lesions and CSF inflammatory mediators in different disease phenotypes, which potentially plays an important role in determining future targeting treatments.

Attempting to reduce the gap between macroscopic and microscopic tissue and lesional structure, diffusion imaging where MRI signal is sensitive to random motion of water can be a helpful tool. Diffusion tensor imaging (DTI) is the most conventional diffusion imaging technique, and it represents the movement of water in a single three-dimensional tensor, however, it does not take into account the heterogeneity in tissue characteristics which in turn influences the reliability of the derived indices. This in turn paved the way for newer multicompartmental diffusion techniques which consider the heterogeneity of tissue compartments. Neurite orientation dispersion and density imaging (NODDI) is a novel diffusion imaging technique that models the CSF space as isotropic volume fraction V_{iso}, while the dendrites and axons are represented as apparent intra-axonal volume fraction V_{in}, and the orientation dispersion ODI, which is a measure of how nonparallel axons disperse about a central orientation providing a cylindrically symmetric Watson distribution [63]. NODDI offered higher sensitivity over other diffusion imaging methods in particular DTI, and especially V_{in} and ODI provide more contrast than other indices which offers helpful insight into MS pathology in the spinal cord as well as microstructural damage in normal-appearing white matter tissue, which does not show any particular abnormality in anatomical scans. It can also provide a valuable monitoring technique to observe tissue evolution even before lesions appearance [63]. However, registration of those sequences to anatomical sequences can pose difficulty.

Magnetic resonance spectroscopy (^{1}H-MRS) of the brain offered insight into the microstructural lesional and extralesional component beyond the macroscopic tissue damage via quantifying different metabolites. However, such application in the spinal cord has been technically challenging until recent years. ^{1}H-MRS is shown to be a good marker of early neuronal loss indicated by lower concentrations of total N-acetyl-aspartate (tNAA), which reflects neuroaxonal integrity, and glutamate-glutamine (Glx), which is a marker of neuronal integrity, in the upper cervical cord of patients with early PPMS even before the development of atrophy. Furthermore, tNAA concentration was lowest in lesional tissue and still affected, but to far less degree, in the normal-appearing tissue when compared with controls. Similarly, Glx concentration was also reduced in spinal cord lesions, likely reflecting axonal degeneration; but levels did not correlate to tNAA which suggests they reflect different pathological processes. On the other hand, both markers showed a good correlation with disability progression in PPMS patients [64].

Magnetization transfer ratio (MTR) is a semi-quantitative technique that provides an indirect estimate of the degree of demyelination and axonal loss, by measuring the magnetization exchange between freely mobile water protons and immobile macromolecular protons. MTR values were found to be significantly lower in cervical spinal cord of early MS patients in comparison with controls even in the absence of spinal cord atrophy; and the same was found in normal-appearing cord tissue which reflects the microstructural demyelination and axonal loss in normal-appearing tissue which should be taken into account in trials developing targeted disease-modifying treatment [65].

A novel approach that showed higher sensitivity to tissue myelin content than conventional MTI is inhomogeneous magnetization transfer imaging. It was proven to be more sensitive to microstructural spinal cord damage in comparison with DTI especially in normal-appearing cord tissue [66]. However, this technique was not compared directly to other myelin-specific imaging techniques such as quantitative MT imaging or myelin water fraction.

Despite the significant contribution of spinal cord imaging to the diagnosis and prognosis of MS, it still faces major technical challenges with a higher likelihood of artifacts due to the cord being a narrow mobile structure, low signal-to-noise ratio, pulse and respiratory-related artifacts, and the lack of normative data. Gray matter disease in the spinal cord as a separate significant entity and its contribution to the disease course has been under-covered due to challenges in imaging acquisition.

With continuous advances in imaging techniques and with the increasing incorporation of higher magnetic field imaging into clinical practice, examining spinal cord gray matter will be feasible. This is in addition to further advances in diffusion and magnetization transfer imaging to help bridge the gap between imaging and pathology and provide a promising biomarker for clinical trials.

14. Conclusion

Understanding disability accumulation is the corner stone of effective management in MS patients. The greatest proportion of disability accumulation is not accounted for by new lesions or relapses hence the term PIRA. The availability of ultra-high-field imaging allowed further exploration of factors associated with PIRA to facilitate the development of targeted disease-modifying treatments in MS. Cortical lesion load contributes to the degree of disability and they need to be taken into consideration during treatment decision-making. Similarly, white matter iron rim lesions frequency is a significant prognostic factor in MS patients, with studies showing that patients who had more than four lesions were more likely to experience future worsening disability. However, this worsening degree of disability was rendered to the higher degree of tissue loss in some iron rim lesions and their evolution into slowly expanding lesions. Further elucidation of the extent of association between those factors and future disability is crucial for the potential evolution of biomarkers to facilitate the development of targeted disease-modifying treatments in MS clinical trials.

Author details

Rasha Abdel-Fahim
Nottingham University Hospitals, Nottingham, UK

*Address all correspondence to: rasha.fahim@doctors.org.uk

References

[1] Kidd D, Barkhof F, McConnell R, Algra PR, Allen IV, Revesz T. Cortical lesions in multiple sclerosis. Brain. 1999;**122**(1):17-26

[2] Calabrese M, Gallo P. Magnetic resonance evidence of cortical onset of multiple sclerosis. Multi Sclerosis Houndmills Basingstoke England. 2009;**15**(8):933-941

[3] Peterson JW, Bö L, Mörk S, Chang A, Trapp BD. Transected neurites, apoptotic neurons, and reduced inflammation in cortical multiple sclerosis lesions. Annals of Neurology. 2001;**50**(3):389-400

[4] Bø L, Vedeler CA, Nyland H, Trapp BD, Mørk SJ. Intracortical multiple sclerosis lesions are not associated with increased lymphocyte infiltration. Multi Sclerosis Houndmills Basingstoke England. 2003;**9**(4):323-331

[5] Abdel-Fahim R, Mistry N, Mougin O, Blazejewska A, Pitiot A, Retkute R, et al. Improved detection of focal cortical lesions using 7T magnetisation transfer imaging in patients with multiple sclerosis. Multiple Sclerosis and Related Disorders. 2014;**3**(2):258-265

[6] Beck ES, Maranzano J, Luciano NJ, Parvathaneni P, Filippini S, Morrison M, et al. Cortical lesion hotspots and association of subpial lesions with disability in multiple sclerosis. Multi Sclerosis Houndmills Basingstoke England. 2022;**28**(9):1351-1363

[7] Trapp BD, Vignos M, Dudman J, Chang A, Fisher E, Staugaitis SM, et al. Cortical neuronal densities and cerebral white matter demyelination in multiple sclerosis: A retrospective study. Lancet Neurology. 2018;**17**(10):870-884

[8] Beck ES, Sati P, Sethi V, Kober T, Dewey B, Bhargava P, et al. Improved visualization of cortical lesions in multiple sclerosis using 7T MP2RAGE. AJNR. American Journal of Neuroradiology. 2018;**39**(3):459-466

[9] Nielsen AS, Kinkel RP, Tinelli E, Benner T, Cohen-Adad J, Mainero C. Focal cortical lesion detection in multiple sclerosis: 3 tesla DIR versus 7 tesla FLASH-T2*. Journal of Magnetic Resonance Imaging. 2012;**35**(3):537-542

[10] Pitt D, Boster A, Pei W, Wohleb E, Jasne A, Zachariah CR, et al. Imaging cortical lesions in multiple sclerosis with ultra-high-field magnetic resonance imaging. Archives of Neurology. 2010;**67**(7):812-818

[11] Kilsdonk ID, Jonkman LE, Klaver R, van Veluw SJ, Zwanenburg JJM, Kuijer JPA, et al. Increased cortical grey matter lesion detection in multiple sclerosis with 7 T MRI: A post-mortem verification study. Brain: A Journal of Neurology. 2016;**139**(Pt 5):1472-1481

[12] Treaba CA, Herranz E, Barletta VT, Mehndiratta A, Ouellette R, Sloane JA, et al. The relevance of multiple sclerosis cortical lesions on cortical thinning and their clinical impact as assessed by 7.0-T MRI. Journal of Neurology. 2021;**268**(7):2473-2481

[13] Nielsen AS, Kinkel RP, Madigan N, Tinelli E, Benner T, Mainero C. Contribution of cortical lesion subtypes at 7T MRI to physical and cognitive performance in MS. Neurology. 2013;**81**(7):641-649

[14] Calabrese M, Poretto V, Favaretto A, Alessio S, Bernardi V, Romualdi C, et al. Cortical lesion load associates with

progression of disability in multiple sclerosis. Brain. 2012;**135**(10):2952-2961

[15] Fartaria MJ, Sati P, Todea A, Radue EW, Rahmanzadeh R, O'Brien K, et al. Automated detection and segmentation of multiple sclerosis lesions using ultra-high-field MP2RAGE. Investigative Radiology 2019;54(6):356-364.

[16] La Rosa F, Beck ES, Abdulkadir A, Thiran JP, Reich DS, Sati P, et al. Automated detection of cortical lesions in multiple sclerosis patients with 7T MRI. In: Martel AL, Abolmaesumi P, Stoyanov D, Mateus D, Zuluaga MA, Zhou SK, et al., editors. Medical Image Computing and Computer Assisted Intervention – MICCAI 2020. Cham: Springer International Publishing; 2020. pp. 584-593

[17] La Rosa F, Beck ES, Maranzano J, Todea RA, van Gelderen P, de Zwart JA, et al. Multiple sclerosis cortical lesion detection with deep learning at ultra-high-field MRI. NMR in Biomedicine. 2022;**35**(8):e4730

[18] University of California, San Francisco MS-EPIC Team, BAC C, Hollenbach JA, Bove R, Kirkish G, Sacco S, et al. Silent progression in disease activity-free relapsing multiple sclerosis. Annals of Neurology. 2019 May;**85**(5):653-666

[19] Weinshenker BG, Bass B, Rice GP, Noseworthy J, Carriere W, Baskerville J, et al. The natural history of multiple sclerosis: A geographically based study. 2. Predictive value of the early clinical course. Brain. Journal of Neurology. 1989;**112**(Pt 6):1419-1428

[20] Kappos L, Wolinsky JS, Giovannoni G, Arnold DL, Wang Q, Bernasconi C, et al. Contribution of relapse-independent progression vs relapse-associated worsening to overall confirmed disability accumulation in typical relapsing multiple sclerosis in a pooled analysis of 2 randomized clinical trials. JAMA Neurology. 2020;**77**(9):1-9

[21] Prosperini L, Ruggieri S, Haggiag S, Tortorella C, Pozzilli C, Gasperini C. Prognostic accuracy of NEDA-3 in long-term outcomes of multiple sclerosis. Neurological Neuroimmunology Neuroinflammation. 2021;**8**(6):e1059

[22] Kappos L, De Stefano N, Freedman MS, Cree BA, Radue EW, Sprenger T, et al. Inclusion of brain volume loss in a revised measure of 'no evidence of disease activity' (NEDA-4) in relapsing-remitting multiple sclerosis. Multi Sclerosis Houndmills Basingstoke England. 2016;**22**(10):1297-1305

[23] Rotstein D, Solomon JM, Sormani MP, Montalban X, Ye XY, Dababneh D, et al. Association of NEDA-4 with No long-term disability progression in multiple sclerosis and comparison with NEDA-3: A systematic review and Meta-analysis. Neurological Neuroimmunology Neuroinflammation. 2022;**9**(6):e200032

[24] Meyer-Moock S, Feng YS, Maeurer M, Dippel FW, Kohlmann T. Systematic literature review and validity evaluation of the expanded disability status scale (EDSS) and the multiple sclerosis functional composite (MSFC) in patients with multiple sclerosis. BMC Neurology. 2014;**14**:58

[25] Noseworthy JH, Vandervoort MK, Wong CJ, Ebers GC. Interrater variability with the expanded disability status scale (EDSS) and functional systems (FS) in a multiple sclerosis clinical trial. Neurology. 1990;**40**(6):971-971

[26] Tiu VE, Enache I, Panea CA, Tiu C, Popescu BO. Predictive MRI biomarkers

in MS-A critical review. Med Kaunas Lith. 2022;**58**(3):377

[27] Pandit L. No evidence of disease activity (NEDA) in multiple sclerosis - shifting the goal posts. Annals of Indian Academy of Neurology. 2019;**22**(3):261-263

[28] Hametner S, Wimmer I, Haider L, Pfeifenbring S, Brück W, Lassmann H. Iron and neurodegeneration in the multiple sclerosis brain. Annals of Neurology. 2013;**74**(6):848-861

[29] Dal-Bianco A, Grabner G, Kronnerwetter C, Weber M, Höftberger R, Berger T, et al. Slow expansion of multiple sclerosis iron rim lesions: Pathology and 7 T magnetic resonance imaging. Acta Neuropathology (Berl). 2017;**133**(1):25-42

[30] Chawla S, Kister I, Wuerfel J, Brisset JC, Liu S, Sinnecker T, et al. Iron and non-Iron-related characteristics of multiple sclerosis and Neuromyelitis Optica lesions at 7T MRI. AJNR. American Journal of Neuroradiology. 2016;**37**(7):1223-1230

[31] Bagnato F, Hametner S, Yao B, van Gelderen P, Merkle H, Cantor FK, et al. Tracking iron in multiple sclerosis: A combined imaging and histopathological study at 7 Tesla. Brain: A Journal of Neurology. 2011;**134**(Pt 12):3602-3615

[32] Prineas JW, Kwon EE, Cho ES, Sharer LR, Barnett MH, Oleszak EL, et al. Immunopathology of secondary-progressive multiple sclerosis. Annals of Neurology. 2001;**50**(5):646-657

[33] Chawla S, Kister I, Sinnecker T, Wuerfel J, Brisset JC, Paul F, et al. Longitudinal study of multiple sclerosis lesions using ultra-high field (7T) multiparametric MR imaging. PLoS One. 2018;**13**(9):e0202918

[34] Sica A, Mantovani A. Macrophage plasticity and polarization: in vivo veritas. The Journal of Clinical Investigation. 2012;**122**(3):787-795

[35] Yao B, Hametner S, van Gelderen P, Merkle H, Chen C, Lassmann H, et al. 7 tesla magnetic resonance imaging to detect cortical pathology in multiple sclerosis. PLoS One. 2014;**9**(10):e108863

[36] Castellaro M, Magliozzi R, Palombit A, Pitteri M, Silvestri E, Camera V, et al. Heterogeneity of cortical lesion susceptibility mapping in multiple sclerosis. AJNR. American Journal of Neuroradiology. 2017;**38**(6):1087-1095

[37] Frischer JM, Weigand SD, Guo Y, Kale N, Parisi JE, Pirko I, et al. Clinical and pathological insights into the dynamic nature of the white matter multiple sclerosis plaque. Annals of Neurology. 2015;**78**(5):710-721

[38] Dal-Bianco A, Grabner G, Kronnerwetter C, Weber M, Kornek B, Kasprian G, et al. Long-term evolution of multiple sclerosis iron rim lesions in 7 T MRI. Brain: A Journal of Neurology. 2021;**144**(3):833-847

[39] Bian W, Harter K, Hammond-Rosenbluth KE, Lupo JM, Xu D, Kelley DA, et al. A serial in vivo 7T magnetic resonance phase imaging study of white matter lesions in multiple sclerosis. Multiple Sclerosis Journal. 2013;**19**(1):69-75

[40] Absinta M, Sati P, Schindler M, Leibovitch EC, Ohayon J, Wu T, et al. Persistent 7-tesla phase rim predicts poor outcome in new multiple sclerosis patient lesions. The Journal of Clinical Investigation. 2016;**126**(7):2597-2609

[41] Elliott C, Wolinsky JS, Hauser SL, Kappos L, Barkhof F, Bernasconi C, et al. Slowly expanding/evolving lesions

as a magnetic resonance imaging marker of chronic active multiple sclerosis lesions. Multi Sclerosis Houndmills Basingstoke England. 2019;**25**(14):1915-1925

[42] Bramow S, Frischer JM, Lassmann H, Koch-Henriksen N, Lucchinetti CF, Sørensen PS, et al. Demyelination versus remyelination in progressive multiple sclerosis. Brain: A Journal of Neurology. 2010;**133**(10):2983-2998

[43] Marques JP, Kober T, Krueger G, van der Zwaag W, Van de Moortele PF, Gruetter R. MP2RAGE, a self bias-field corrected sequence for improved segmentation and T1-mapping at high field. NeuroImage. 2010;**49**(2):1271-1281

[44] Kolb H, Absinta M, Beck ES, Ha SK, Song Y, Norato G, et al. 7T MRI differentiates Remyelinated from demyelinated multiple sclerosis lesions. Annals of Neurology. 2021;**90**(4):612-626

[45] Patrikios P, Stadelmann C, Kutzelnigg A, Rauschka H, Schmidbauer M, Laursen H, et al. Remyelination is extensive in a subset of multiple sclerosis patients. Brain: A Journal of Neurology. 2006;**129**(Pt 12):3165-3172

[46] Franklin RJ, Blakemore WF. To what extent is oligodendrocyte progenitor migration a limiting factor in the remyelination of multiple sclerosis lesions? Multiple Sclerosis Journal. 1997;**3**(2):84-87

[47] Preziosa P, Pagani E, Meani A, Moiola L, Rodegher M, Filippi M, et al. Slowly expanding lesions predict 9-year multiple sclerosis disease progression. Neurological Neuroimmunological Neuroinflammation. 2022;**9**(2):e1139

[48] Altokhis AI, Hibbert AM, Allen CM, Mougin O, Alotaibi A, Lim SY, et al. Longitudinal clinical study of patients with iron rim lesions in multiple sclerosis. Multi Sclerosis Houndmills Basingstoke England. 2022;**24**:1352

[49] Preziosa P, Pagani E, Moiola L, Rodegher M, Filippi M, Rocca MA. Occurrence and microstructural features of slowly expanding lesions on fingolimod or natalizumab treatment in multiple sclerosis. Multiple Sclerosis Journal. 2021;**27**(10):1520-1532

[50] Calvi A, Tur C, Chard D, Stutters J, Ciccarelli O, Cortese R, et al. Slowly expanding lesions relate to persisting black-holes and clinical outcomes in relapse-onset multiple sclerosis. NeuroImage Clinic. 2022;**35**:103048

[51] Elliott C, Belachew S, Wolinsky JS, Hauser SL, Kappos L, Barkhof F, et al. Chronic white matter lesion activity predicts clinical progression in primary progressive multiple sclerosis. Brain: A Journal of Neurology. 2019;**142**(9):2787-2799

[52] Elliott C, Arnold DL, Chen H, Ke C, Zhu L, Chang I, et al. Patterning chronic active demyelination in slowly expanding/evolving white matter MS lesions. AJNR. American Journal of Neuroradiology. 2020;**41**(9):1584-1591

[53] Barkhof F, Calabresi PA, Miller DH, Reingold SC. Imaging outcomes for neuroprotection and repair in multiple sclerosis trials. Nature Reviews. Neurology. 2009;**5**(5):256-266

[54] Geisseler O, Pflugshaupt T, Bezzola L, Reuter K, Weller D, Schuknecht B, et al. The relevance of cortical lesions in patients with multiple sclerosis. BMC Neurology. 2016;**16**(1):204

[55] Sastre-Garriga J, Ingle GT, Chard DT, Ramió-Torrentà L, Miller DH, Thompson AJ. Grey and white matter atrophy in early clinical stages of

primary progressive multiple sclerosis. NeuroImage. 2004;**22**(1):353-359

[56] Mina Y, Azodi S, Dubuche T, Andrada F, Osuorah I, Ohayon J, et al. Cervical and thoracic cord atrophy in multiple sclerosis phenotypes: Quantification and correlation with clinical disability. NeuroImage Clinic. 2021;**30**:102680

[57] Bussas M, El Husseini M, Harabacz L, Pineker V, Grahl S, Pongratz V, et al. Multiple sclerosis lesions and atrophy in the spinal cord: Distribution across vertebral levels and correlation with disability. NeuroImage Clinic. 2022;**34**:103006

[58] Bieniek M, Altmann DR, Davies GR, Ingle GT, Rashid W, Sastre-Garriga J, et al. Cord atrophy separates early primary progressive and relapsing remitting multiple sclerosis. Journal of Neurology, Neurosurgery, and Psychiatry. 2006;**77**(9):1036-1039

[59] Prados F, Moccia M, Johnson A, Yiannakas M, Grussu F, Cardoso MJ, et al. Generalised boundary shift integral for longitudinal assessment of spinal cord atrophy. NeuroImage. 2020;**209**:116489

[60] Eden D, Gros C, Badji A, Dupont SM, De Leener B, Maranzano J, et al. Spatial distribution of multiple sclerosis lesions in the cervical spinal cord. Brain: A Journal of Neurology. 2019;**142**(3):633-646

[61] Lassmann H. Pathogenic mechanisms associated with different clinical courses of multiple sclerosis. Frontiers in Immunology. 2018;**9**:3116

[62] Ouellette R, Treaba CA, Granberg T, Herranz E, Barletta V, Mehndiratta A, et al. 7 T imaging reveals a gradient in spinal cord lesion distribution in multiple sclerosis. Brain: A Journal of Neurology. 2020;**143**(10):2973-2987

[63] By S, Xu J, Box BA, Bagnato FR, Smith SA. Application and evaluation of NODDI in the cervical spinal cord of multiple sclerosis patients. NeuroImage Clinic. 2017;**15**:333-342

[64] Abdel-Aziz K, Schneider T, Solanky BS, Yiannakas MC, Altmann DR, Wheeler-Kingshott CAM, et al. Evidence for early neurodegeneration in the cervical cord of patients with primary progressive multiple sclerosis. Brain: A Journal of Neurology. 2015;**138**(Pt 6): 1568-1582

[65] Combès B, Kerbrat A, Ferré JC, Callot V, Maranzano J, Badji A, et al. Focal and diffuse cervical spinal cord damage in patients with early relapsing–remitting MS: A multicentre magnetisation transfer ratio study. Multiple Sclerosis Journal. 2019;**25**(8):1113-1123

[66] Rasoanandrianina H, Demortière S, Trabelsi A, Ranjeva JP, Girard O, Duhamel G, et al. Sensitivity of the inhomogeneous magnetization transfer imaging technique to spinal cord damage in multiple sclerosis. AJNR. American Journal of Neuroradiology. 2020;**41**(5):929-937